THE
ORGANIC
BABY FOOD
BOOK

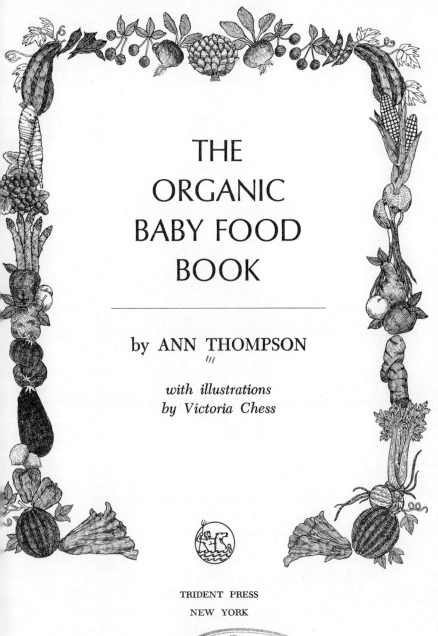

THE
ORGANIC
BABY FOOD
BOOK

by ANN THOMPSON

*with illustrations
by Victoria Chess*

TRIDENT PRESS

NEW YORK

FOR MAX

SBN 671-27107-5
Library of Congress Catalog Card Number: 73-82872
Designed by Irving Perkins
Manufactured in the United States of America

1 2 3 4 5 6 7 8 9 10

40,609

CONTENTS

5

INTRODUCTION

This is an organic baby-food cookbook. The recipes are simple. With the help of an ordinary blender, you can prepare many of them in fifteen minutes or less. True, that healthy baby grinning out at you from the array of brilliantly packaged baby foods at your local market is almost irresistible; what's more, the canned food takes no time at all to open and serve. One would almost believe that the family farm, with its bushels of harvested apples, strings of drying peppers and corn, and rich smell of freshly baked bread is compressed, like an eager genie, into that appealing little jar on the shelf. Don't believe it. The speed and ease of such foods can never compensate for the lack of real food value and the incredible wastes of the packaging industry.

Nutritionists, doctors and health specialists in growing numbers are concerned that the food industry's emphasis on fancy packaging rather than essential nutrients may have seriously undermined the healthfulness of the American diet. This concern is especially serious with respect to the growth and development of infants and young children. Scientists have isolated nutrition as the crucial element in the development of the infant's permanent mental capacities. The message is simple: Learn as much as you can about baby food and learn it before your baby is born.

If we can begin to feed our children the whole good foods of the earth itself, we can help to build a future generation that will have better health, and a more harmonious life with nature and man.

Mother's milk is undoubtedly the best possible food for your infant. I recommend nursing your baby for at least six months, if possible. Many of my friends have continued to nurse their babies for as long as two years or more and the children always seemed hearty, active, and free from many sicknesses. Solid food *does not* need to be introduced before your baby is six months old. Some mothers, however, cannot nurse that long or must be absent from the home for extended periods and wish to introduce semi-solid foods as early as three months. All the recipes in this book are dated with the age at which I began to feed them to my baby. You may want to wait longer to introduce many of these to your child. Others you will want to start a bit earlier than I did. There are no hard-and-fast rules. Consult your own medical authorities and rely on a mother's intuitive knowledge of her own child. Take care to avoid any of those packaged infant formulas. Many hospitals automatically start the babies on them if you don't let them know you want to start with natural foods for your child. There is always some relatively simple formula that can be made up quickly using natural foods. Consult your doctor about this before your child is born.

All of the recipes in this book call for the use of fresh or dried fruits and vegetables. I recommend that whenever possible you get your fruit and vegetables from an organic source. I found it impossible, however, due to the prohibitive prices, to buy entirely at organic food stores. One alternative is to get together with about ten or more people and organize a food co-op to buy at wholesale prices. When you do use produce from a regular market, it's a good idea to scrub it with a vegetable brush and pure soap preparation. You can get a good liquid castile soap in most organic food stores. Try to avoid peeling fruits or vegetables, if you can—you'll peel away the vitamins that are close to the surface. Some produce, however, particularly apples, cucumbers and turnips, is often waxed to present a more appealing surface. While it may look glossy and sleek, wax isn't good for you and it should be peeled away.

Dried fruits are always good to use, particularly if you're a busy mother or one who must travel frequently, as they keep for long periods of time with no special equipment. They also make a great "sweet treat" to give children in place of commercially manufactured candy. During the winter, in many areas, fresh produce is of poor quality with very little variety. Fruits and vegetables ripen in shipping crates instead of on the trees, which robs them of vitamins. You can fill out your diet during such times with dried fruits. It's very important to get dried fruits from an organic source, if at all possible. Most commercially prepared dried fruits are heavily sulphured. Always try to use the fresh fruits and vegetables that are grown close to you. It gives you a much better chance of getting vine-ripened produce.

One thing to keep in mind while reading this cookbook, or any other, is that recipes are only approximations of the quantity of the various ingredients. Once you've cooked a recipe and understand it better, never hesitate to experiment and make changes. If you find the consistency of the baby foods in Chapters III and IV either too solid or too runny for your baby's tastes, alter by adding yogurt to thicken or juice to liquefy. I have tried to structure these recipes very loosely so that they can lend themselves to variations. I believe they can be the basis of a sound diet for a baby, and I encourage mothers to experiment with them and broaden the range set down here. You will find a list of the principal vitamins and minerals present at the end of each recipe. This is by no means a complete listing, as I have only mentioned the vitamins and minerals present in some amount. The recipes contain other vitamins and minerals in less significant amounts. I have also included a bibliography of recommended readings. They represent a wide range of recipes and views within the world of organic cooking. Many I do not entirely agree with, but all have helped me in some manner to find my own way with food.

It is possible to have a healthy, well-balanced diet without the use of meat. Soybeans, particularly, are emerging as the best plant source of protein, with protein amounts equivalent to that obtained from meat. This ancient, humble bean is in so many ways the most valuable of all plant foods. Modern food technology, in its race with famine and the population growth, is more and more concerned with research into soybean uses. Soybeans contain all the essential amino acids, practically all the known vitamins, high-quality protein, lecithin, calcium, phosphorus and iron. They lend themselves to almost infinite variations; they can become bean sprouts, milk, cheese, curd, a meatlike pulp, butter, sauces, flour, bread, and other foods. Amazing but true. This bean is bound to become a most important food of the future. Protein for a vegetarian diet is also derived from the whole grains of all cereals, especially the bran and germ. Nuts, seeds, and yeast are also good sources of protein. Milk products are excellent. As a young baby, my son especially loved yogurt, either in his bottle as a plain drink or blended with other juices (see Chapter IV). Yogurt is delicious combined with grains, fruits or vegetables. Cottage cheese and soft cheeses made from milk, such as Muenster, are also good first cheeses for a baby.

One must also consider the quality of the meat in the average diet. Most animals today are raised in crowded concentrations, not in the idyllic pastoral farm scene of days gone by. In heavy cattle-producing areas, animals are crowded into small, tight feedlots, and the stench of manure fills the air of whole counties. In this unhealthful atmosphere animals are often bolstered up with antibiotics, hormones and feed which contains traces of DDT.

"Food technologists" or "food engineers" in this country are generally agreed that the future will bring too many more Americans for the animal protein now available. Some have suggested that we might next focus our gaze on the blue whale as a source of animal protein, but we have already decimated that species.

Future Americans will undoubtedly have to face some kind of a reduction in their consumption of meat. Now is definitely the time to think about some kind of change. If you don't want to cut meat from your diet entirely, just begin to experiment with a few meals a week that put the central focus on beans, grains, cheese, nuts, or other non-meat foods. I hope this book will show you some interesting ways to do this from the birth of your child through the years of family life.

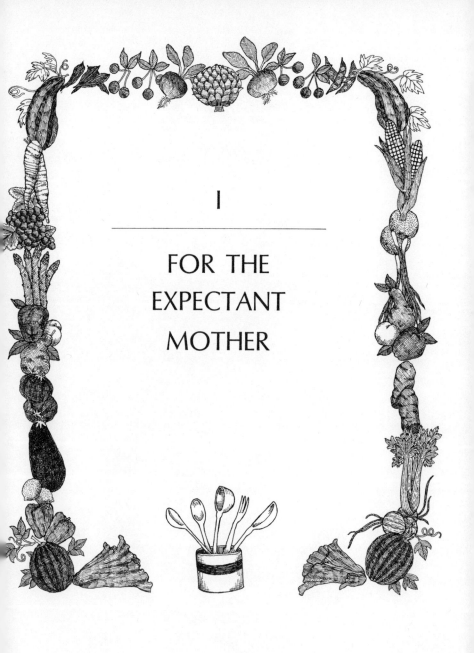

I

FOR THE
EXPECTANT
MOTHER

Treat yourself right before and during your pregnancy. Eat well, exercise daily and get enough sleep. Nutritionally, the baby depends totally on what your body supplies. How well you can supply your child's needs and preserve your own good health depends on the state of your own body when you conceive. Organic baby feeding begins with organic girl feeding long before conception.

The following are just a few recipes that could be included in your diet as a part of good prenatal care.

A Wonderful Body Oil

Vegetable oil applied lightly to the body helps to increase the benefits from the sun, and in pregnancy it aids suppleness of breasts and abdominal area. Oil should not be applied undiluted to the skin, but rubbed on from a large swab of cotton wool previously dampened in plain water; or water with a few drops of vinegar added is better, and buttermilk is excellent instead of water. It is easy to collect fragrant flowers and leaves, pound them into pulp and add them to the oils and infuse them in glass bottles or jars, well-stoppered, in sunlight or in a warm oven. When hot sun is available, it is preferable to stand the bottles in a container of sand. This attracts and holds the sun-heat. Use about two tablespoons of flowers, and/or leaves, to every pint of oil, add also a dessertspoon of vinegar per pint of oil to help break up the plant matter. Herbs which I use most, are sprigs of garden lavender, rosemary, southernwood and wild meadowsweet, woodruff, elder-blossom, briar-rose, gorse.

—JULIETTE DE BAIRACLI LEVY
Nature's Children, page 15

Rub this daily into your breasts and abdomen as a guard against stretch marks. Cocoa butter can also be used for this purpose.

Daily Breakfast Drink

½ cup goat's-milk yogurt*
½ cup fresh orange juice
⅓ ripe banana
1 tablespoon brewer's yeast
1 tablespoon blackstrap molasses
1 tablespoon raw wheat germ

Combine all ingredients in blender and purée until light and frothy. This is good to drink every day of your pregnancy because of its high protein, calcium and iron content. Drink at breakfast or in the early afternoon. 1 serving.

Contains protein, calcium, iron, vitamins A, B, C and E.

* Cow's-milk yogurt may be substituted, but goat's is preferable.

Between Meals

1 cup fresh orange juice
2 tablespoons cottage cheese
2 calcium lactate tablets
1 teaspoon tupelo honey

Combine all ingredients in blender and liquefy until frothy. 1 serving.
This is an easy once-a-day drink for extra protein and calcium that you may need during your pregnancy.

Contains protein, calcium, vitamins A, B and C.

Bel Paese Soufflé

1 cup soybeans, cooked and puréed
1 Spanish onion, finely grated
½ teaspoon ground sage
½ teaspoon sea salt
3 tablespoons safflower oil

3 tablespoons wholewheat flour
1 cup hot milk
½ cup Bel Paese* cheese, grated and tightly packed
4 egg yolks, beaten
4 egg whites, beaten stiff

Preheat oven to 300° F.

In a large mixing bowl, combine puréed soybeans, grated onion, sage and salt.

Heat oil in a heavy saucepan and blend in flour with a wire whisk. Add the milk slowly, stirring constantly. Add the cheese and continue to cook over a low flame, stirring constantly until thickened. Remove from heat and combine with soybean mixture.

When mixture cools, blend in egg yolks and fold in egg whites. Turn into a buttered soufflé dish or 6 custard cups. Place cooking dish or custard cups in a large shallow baking pan with about 1 inch hot water in it. Cook soufflé for about 50 to 60 minutes, or until firm and nicely browned on top. If custard cups are used, cook for about 35 minutes. 4 servings.

This makes a lovely light soufflé, very good to eat often for lunch or dinner during pregnancy. Serve with a tossed vegetable salad and some yogurt and fruit for dessert. This is also an excellent first food for your baby—start at 6 months.

Contains protein, iron, calcium, lecithin, phosphorous, vitamins A, B and C.

* If Bel Paese cheese is not available, use sharp Cheddar, Gouda, or a combination of both.

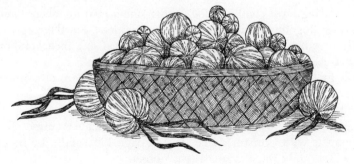

Mama's Stuffed Peppers

    4 large green peppers
    2 tablespoons lemon juice
    5 tablespoons safflower oil
    1 clove garlic, minced
    1 large Spanish onion, chopped
 2½ tablespoons blackstrap molasses
 2½ tablespoons Tamari soy sauce
   ¼ cup celery
   ¼ cup green pepper, chopped
    1 cup Steamed Brown Rice (page 42)
    1 cup Cooked Lentils (page 43)
   ⅔ cup Cheddar cheese, tightly packed
   ⅔ cup walnuts, chopped
   ½ cup vegetable bouillon or mixture of Tamari soy sauce and
      water

Preheat oven to 350° F.

Wash the peppers and cut off the stem end; remove the veins and seeds and rub the insides with lemon juice.

Heat the oil in a skillet and add garlic; sauté until garlic is slightly browned and add onion. Continue to sauté until onions are wilted and slightly brown, about 15 minutes. Add a bit of water to keep them moist, if necessary. Stir in molasses and soy sauce and cook for about 30 seconds. Add celery and pepper and continue to cook for about 6 to 8 minutes, or until pepper and celery are just cooked.

In a mixing bowl combine rice, lentils, onion mixture, cheese and nuts. Toss together well and stuff into peppers. Fit the peppers closely together in a baking dish and add about one inch bouillon or soy sauce-water mixture.

Bake for about 35 to 40 minutes and then sprinkle tops of peppers with cheese and let bake a few minutes more, or until cheese begins to melt. 4 servings.

This is another example of a good lunch or dinner entrée. Try the peppers with Christmas Eve Beans (page 140) and a bottle of hearty Burgundy for a winter-night dinner.

Contains protein, iron, calcium, lecithin, phosphorus, vitamins A, B, C and E.

Asian Garden Salad

2 tablespoons safflower oil
1 clove garlic, minced
1 cup fresh mushrooms, sliced
2 tablespoons Tamari soy sauce
1 cup Steamed Brown Rice (page 42)
1 cup cooked Hijiki Sea Vegetable (page 142)
⅔ cup mung beans sprouts
⅓ cup parsley, finely minced
3 tablespoons sunflower seeds
¼ cup safflower oil
¼ cup fresh lemon or lime juice

Heat two tablespoons of oil in skillet and add garlic. Sauté until garlic is slightly browned and add mushrooms; sauté 3 to 5 minutes, or until mushrooms are just cooked. Add Tamari soy sauce during last minute of cooking. Set aside to cool.

Combine rice, seaweed, sprouts, parsley, and seeds in a salad bowl and toss well. Add mushrooms and pan juices.

Combine oil and lemon or lime juice. Pour over salad and toss well. Season with more Tamari if desired. 3 or 4 servings.

This is a fine salad to eat often when you are pregnant. Its high amounts of iron and protein make it a good regular item in your diet.

Contains protein, calcium, lecithin, phosphorous, iron, vitamins A, B, C and E.

A Yogurt Dessert

    6 dried apricots
      Apricot nectar to cover
    3 teaspoons tupelo honey
    1 cup yogurt
    ¼ cup raw wheat germ
    ½ cup fresh pineapple chunks
    ½ cup fresh strawberries
    ⅓ cup walnuts, chopped
      Tupelo honey to taste

Soak apricots in nectar overnight to soften and plump up. Pour apricots, any extra juice and honey into blender and purée to a heavy paste.

In a mixing bowl combine yogurt, wheat germ and apricot paste. Stir together well. Add fruit and fold in. Sprinkle with walnuts and top with a little more honey. 2 servings.

When your sweet cravings drive you mad, whip up this dessert and eat away, knowing that you're getting your vitamins' worth.

Contains protein, calcium, iron, vitamins A, B, C and E.

See Chapter V for many more good pregnancy foods.

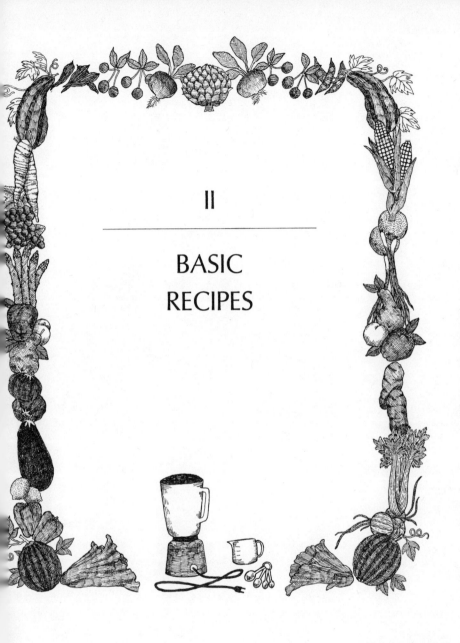

II

BASIC
RECIPES

YOGURT AND MILK

Yogurt

1 tablespoon yogurt culture*
1 quart skim milk (or raw milk or goat's milk)
3 to 4 heaping tablespoons nonfat dried milk

Place milk (your choice) in saucepan and add dried milk. Stir well with wire whisk until completely dissolved; heat milk to the boiling point, but do not allow to boil. Remove from heat and let cool to lukewarm.

Put tablespoon of yogurt culture in a cup and add about 4 or 5 tablespoons of lukewarm milk; stir until completely dissolved and pour back into lukewarm milk. Stir well with wire whisk.

Pour milk into yogurt maker or thermos bottle and allow to sit in a warm, draft-free place for about 7 or 8 hours. 4 servings.

VARIATION: Add a vanilla bean or a tablespoon of honey to yogurt before placing in yogurt maker for a delightful, subtle flavor variation.

Contains protein, calcium, phosphorous, vitamins A and B.

---

* To start your original yogurt culture, use either one tablespoon of commercial yogurt or a packaged dry yogurt culture, which organic food stores sometimes stock. After you have made your first batch of yogurt, save one tablespoon to make the next batch and so on.

Soybean Milk

>   2 teaspoons raisins
>   Apple juice to cover
>   1 teaspoon honey
>   4 cups water
>   1 cup soybean powder

Soften raisins overnight in apple juice in refrigerator. Put raisins and excess juice in the blender. Add honey and water, then soybean powder. Make sure the soybean powder is put on top of the water to facilitate blending. Liquefy in the blender at high speed until thoroughly mixed. You can give this to a baby in place of regular cow's milk. 1 quart.

Contains protein, calcium, iron, lecithin, phosphorus, potassium and vitamins A and B.

Dried Milk

>   6 heaping tablespoons spray-dried milk
>   4 cups water

Combine dried milk and water and mix in blender. You can give this to a baby in place of regular cow's milk. 1 quart.

VARIATION: Add more dried milk for a richer drink, or a teaspoonful of honey for every quart made.

Contains protein, calcium, phosphorus, potassium, sodium and vitamins A and B.

CEREALS AND BREADS

Abby Van Derek's Incredible Granola (the best)

>   4 cups rolled oats
>   1 cup rolled rye
>   1 cup rolled wheat

    1 cup wheat germ
    ½ cup sesame seeds
    ½ cup sunflower seeds
    ½ cup chopped cashews
    ½ cup almonds
    ½ cup chopped pecans
    ½ cup whole pine nuts
    ½ cup unsweetened shredded coconut
    2½ teaspoons sea salt
    ¼ cup corn oil
    ½ cup tupelo honey
    1 cup raisins
    1 cup chopped dried apples
    1 cup pitted and chopped apricots

Combine all ingredients except dried fruits. Mix together thoroughly and lay out on a cookie sheet. Roast at 350° F. Keep turning until done, about 45 minutes. Remove from oven and let cool; keep turning while cereal cools to avoid sticking together. When cool, add raisins, apples and apricots. Store in glass jars in a cool place. About 30 servings.

Serve from 6 months on. Just add milk, also some fresh fruit if you wish. Let stand a few minutes and then purée in blender. Serve as is to the whole family for breakfast.

Contains protein, calcium, phosphorus, potassium, sodium, niacin, vitamins A, B and C.

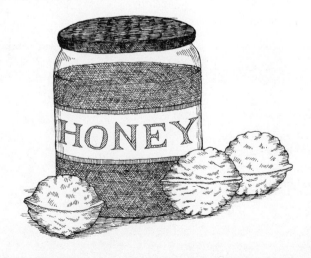

Basic Cereal for Baby

½ cup sesame seeds
1 cup almonds
½ cup wheat germ
3 cups rolled oats
¼ cup safflower oil
¼ cup honey
   Water to moisten

Put some sesame seeds and almonds through a grinder until a powdery texture is achieved. Mix together with wheat germ and oats. Add oil and honey and enough water to barely moisten all ingredients and toss very well. Spread evenly on a cookie sheet and bake in a slow oven (about 300° F.) for 45 minutes to 1 hour, or until lightly browned and somewhat crunchy. 10 to 15 servings.

Serve from 3 months on. Begin with a couple of tablespoons and observe how well the baby digests it; increase quantity from that point on. To serve a small baby, mix ⅓ cup cereal with ⅓ cup yogurt and enough milk to moisten well. Allow mixture to sit about ½ hour before serving time to insure a soft enough texture for baby to digest, or run it through the blender for a few seconds. You can also mix in some fruit or vegetable purée (suggestions in Chapter III) as the baby begins to take more fruits and vegetables. When the baby has enough teeth, you can begin to use whole sesame seeds and almond chunks, raisins, walnut pieces, dried or fresh fruits, etc.

Contains iron, calcium, phosphorus, potassium and vitamin B.

Hunza Breakfast

1 cup wheatberries
1 cup buckwheat
1 cup rye
1 cup barley

1 cup oat groats
1 cup millet
1 cup sesame seeds
1 cup lentils
1 cup brown rice
1 cup flax
1 cup alfalfa seeds
1 cup almonds
1 cup cashews

Mix all ingredients and store in a very cool cellar or in your refrigerator. At night take 3 or 4 tablespoons of the mixture per serving and grind it in a blender or electric seed mill. Cover with water and let stand at room temperature. In the morning, add your own choice of fresh fruits, honey and milk. For a baby, you may want to run the entire mixture through the blender again before serving. Makes 50 to 60 servings.

Serve from 6 months on. This is a very fine breakfast food for the entire family.

Contains protein, iron, calcium, phosphorus, potassium, niacin, sodium, vitamins A, B and E.

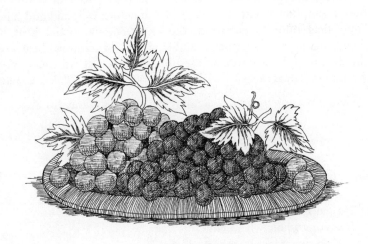

Hush-a-bye, baby, lie still with thy daddy,
Thy mammy is gone to the mill
To get some meal to bake a bread
So pray, my dear baby, lie still.

—MOTHER GOOSE

The Gilded Carriage's Herb Bread

```
  3  cups whole wheat flour
  3  cups unbleached white flour
  2  teaspoons yeast (cake or dry)
2½  cups warm water
 ¼  cup soft butter
  4  teaspoons sea salt
 ¼  cup honey
2½  teaspoons caraway seeds
  1  teaspoon nutmeg
  1  teaspoon sage
  1  teaspoon dill weed
```

Sift the 2 flours together. Dissolve the yeast in warm water. Add butter, salt, honey and seasonings. Stir together well and add 3 cups flour. Beat until smooth. Add the remaining flour and beat. Let dough rise in the bowl until double, about 45 minutes. Beat down the dough, and place in 2 greased bread pans. Let rise again, about 45 minutes. Bake at 375° F. for 40 to 50 minutes. Makes 2 loaves.

Contains protein, iron, calcium, phosphorus, vitamins A and B.

Gig's Dill Bread

```
1¼  cups unbleached white flour
1¼  cups whole wheat flour
  1  teaspoon yeast (cake or dry)
```

¼ cup warm water
1 cup warm cottage cheese
2 teaspoons honey
1 teaspoon butter
1 teaspoon dill seed
1 teaspoon dill weed
1 teaspoon sea salt
¼ teaspoon baking soda
1 egg, well beaten

Sift the flours together. Dissolve yeast in water. Add cottage cheese and stir. Add the rest of the ingredients. Beat well. The dough will be very stiff. Let rise for about 1 hour. Beat down and place in a buttered pan. Butter top of the loaf and bake at 325° F. for 25 minutes; increase heat to 350° for 15 more minutes. Makes 1 loaf.

Contains protein, iron, calcium, phosphorus, vitamins A and B.

Whole Wheat Cuban Bread

4 packages yeast
2½ cups warm water
2 tablespoons sea salt
1½ tablespoons honey
7–8 cups wholewheat flour
½ cup cornmeal
3 tablespoons sesame seeds

Dissolve yeast in ½ cup of the water. Add the rest of the water, the salt and honey. Mix together and add enough flour to make a stiff dough. Knead dough well until it is completely smooth. Place dough in bowl, lightly flour the top, and let it rise until double, about 45 minutes. Punch down; divide into 3 pieces. Shape each into a long sausage by stretching and rolling. Place loaves well apart on a baking sheet that has been sprinkled with the cornmeal. With a knife, slash each loaf a few times across the top. Brush lightly with water and sprinkle with sesame seeds. Place on the lowest rack in a cold oven. Set oven at 350 degrees F. and bake for 1 hour to 65 minutes. Makes 3 loaves.

Serve as soon as your baby begins to teethe. This delicious crusty bread is excellent served warm with soups such as Bengalese Lentil Soup (page 157) or with any winter-night casserole or stew.

Contains protein, calcium, phosphorus, iron, vitamin B.

Whole Wheat Yeast Bread

- ½ cup lukewarm water
- 1 package yeast
- 1 cup goat's milk (or substitute cow's milk)
- ½ cup boiling water
- ¼ cup blackstrap molasses
- 2 teaspoons sea salt
- 3 cups barley flour
- 3 cups whole wheat flour

In a mixing bowl put lukewarm water and yeast. Let stand 5 minutes and then stir. In another bowl combine milk, boiling water, molasses and salt. Stir together well and combine with yeast mixture.

Add 3 cups barley flour and beat very well. Then add whole wheat flour, stirring with a large wooden spoon meanwhile. Knead well.

When smooth, let rise until twice the size (approximately 1 hour). Shape into 2 loaves, place in oiled, lightly floured tins and let rise until double in size, about 45 to 50 minutes.

Bake about 45 to 50 minutes at 375° F. Makes 2 loaves.

Contains protein, iron, calcium, phosphorus, potassium, sodium, vitamin A, B and niacin.

Sesame Bread

- 2 cups whole wheat flour and 1 cup unbleached white flour
      or
- 3 cups unbleached white flour

  1 teaspoon sea salt
2½ teaspoons baking powder
 ½ cup toasted sesame seeds
 ⅔ cup honey
 ¼ cup safflower oil
  2 eggs
  2 teaspoons grated lemon rind
1½ cups milk
  1 tablespoon untoasted sesame seeds

Sift together flour, salt and baking powder. Stir in toasted sesame seeds. Cream the honey and safflower oil until light and well mixed; beat in the eggs. Add lemon rind and milk. Pour into flour mixture all at once and mix only until ingredients are completely blended. Use a rubber spatula to get excess flour away from the edges. Pour into a greased and lightly floured 9x5x3-inch loaf pan. Sprinkle the untoasted sesame seeds on the top and bake for 1 hour and 10 minutes at 350° F. Makes 1 loaf.

Serve from 8 months on. This is good toasted and spread lightly with ricotta or cream cheese for a snack. Use for breakfast toasted and broken into bits with a soft-boiled egg stirred in.

Contains protein, calcium, iron, phosphorus, vitamins A and C.

Banana Nut Bread

1¾ cups sifted whole wheat flour
 ⅔ cup raw sugar
  2 teaspoons baking powder
 ½ teaspoon sea salt
  2 eggs, well beaten
 ¼ cup milk
 ¼ cup safflower oil
  1 cup mashed bananas
 ½ cup ground walnuts
 ½ teaspoon vanilla

Sift dry ingredients together; combine eggs, milk, oil and bananas;

add dry ingredients and beat well. Stir in nuts and vanilla. Pour into a 9x5x3-inch greased and lightly floured loaf pan. Bake at 350° F. for 1 hour, or until done. Makes 1 loaf.

Serve from 6 months. This makes a good breakfast bread for babies. Slice and toast to a golden brown; break into bits and crack a soft-boiled egg over bread. Mix well until bread is soft, and feed.

Contains protein, lecithin, phosphorus, potassium, sodium, niacin, vitamins A, B_{12} and C.

Gig Basil's Pretzels

  1½ cups unbleached white flour
  1½ cups whole wheat flour
   3 teaspoons yeast
   1 cup warm water
   2 teaspoons baking soda
   1 egg, well beaten
     Butter
     Coarse sea salt
     Caraway seeds

Sift flours together; dissolve yeast in water in bowl. Gradually add flours to yeast-water mixture, making a very stiff dough. Knead dough until smooth, about 5 minutes. Grease a large mixing bowl and place dough in it. Butter the top of the dough and let it rise for 30 minutes.

Fill a large pan half full of water, add baking soda and bring to a simmer. After the dough has risen, place it on a board (lightly floured) and roll it into an 8-inch square. Cut it into strips about ½ inch wide. Shape into pretzels—in the shape of the number 8.

Slip the pretzels into the simmering water, one at a time. They will sink, then rise. Remove and place them on a greased cookie sheet about an inch apart. Brush each with beaten egg; sprinkle with salt and caraway seeds. Bake at 400° F. for 15 minutes. Makes 16 pretzels.

Contains protein, iron, phosphorus, vitamins A and B.

Tortillas

    2 cups unbleached white flour
    1 cup cornmeal
    ½ teaspoon sea salt
    2 eggs, well beaten
    3 cups water

Combine all ingredients. Beat throughly. Heat an ungreased griddle or skillet to medium heat. Pour about three tablespoons of batter onto it; when edges look dry, turn the tortillas and cook the other side until completely dry. Makes about 20 tortillas.

Contains protein, iron, calcium, phosphorus, vitamins A and B.

GRAINS AND DRIED BEANS

Oats, peas, beans and barley grows,
How, you nor I, nor nobody knows.
                    —MOTHER GOOSE

A hint about cooking grains and dried beans: All do best with gentle cooking and the least amount of stirring. This helps to keep them unbroken.

Cooked Soybeans

    1 cup soybeans
    4 cups water

Soak soybeans in water overnight in the refrigerator. Next morning bring beans and soaking water to a boil. Cover, reduce heat and let simmer slowly until done, about 2½ hours. 3 or 4 servings.

VARIATION: Add an onion stuck with 2 cloves and a pinch of thyme to the cooking water.

Contains protein, calcium, iron, phosphorus, potassium and vitamins A and B.

Steamed Brown Rice

> 1 cup brown rice
> 2 cups water

Bring 2 cups water to a boil while rinsing rice in cold water. When water boils, add rice and bring again to a full, rolling boil. Cover and reduce flame. Simmer until liquid is evaporated and rice sticks to the bottom of the pot, about 30 minutes. Mix before serving. 2 or 3 servings.

VARIATION: For rice of a more sharply defined grain, good for mixing in salads with fresh vegetables: cook as above for 20 minutes. Then remove lid and turn up flame until liquid is completely evaporated.

Contains protein, calcium, iron, niacin and vitamins A and B.

Mushy Rice for Baby

> 1 cup brown rice
> 3 cups water

Bring 3 cups water to a boil while rinsing rice in cold water. When water boils, add rice and bring again to a full, rolling boil. Cover and reduce flame. Simmer until liquid is evaporated and rice sticks to the bottom of the pot, about 1 hour. Mash with fork or purée in blender before serving. About 5 baby servings.

Contains protein, calcium, phosphorus, niacin, iron and vitamins A and B.

Cooked Rice and Lentils

> Heaping ½ cup brown rice
> Scant ½ cup lentils
> 2 cups water

Rinse rice and lentils together in cold water. Meanwhile bring 2 cups water to a boil. Add to boiling water and reduce heat to a slow simmer. Cover and cook until done, about 35 minutes. 2 or 3 servings.

VARIATION: This combination forms the basis for many very tasty casseroles. Add ingredients such as soy sauce, blackstrap molasses, mushrooms, cheese or nuts.

Contains protein, iron, calcium, phosphorus, potassium, niacin, vitamins A and B.

Cooked Lentils

    2 cups water
    1 cup lentils

Bring water to a boil. Sort and rinse lentils. Add lentils to the boiling water and reduce heat to a slow simmer. Cover and let cook until done, about 35 to 40 minutes. 2 or 3 servings.

VARIATION: For a richer flavor, add a small onion stuck with a clove and one teaspoonful of blackstrap molasses to the cooking water.

Contains protein, iron, calcium, phosphorus, potassium, vitamins A and B.

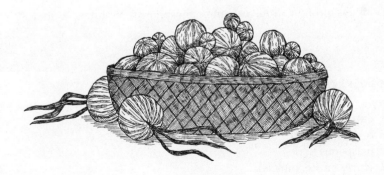

Cooked Millet

½ teaspoon safflower oil
½ cup millet
2 cups boiling water

Heat oil in pot and add millet. Stir millet constantly until it's slightly browned and gives off a nutlike aroma. Add water, cover pot and lower flame. Cook for 30 minutes. 2 servings.

Contains protein, calcium, vitamin A.

Cooked Bulgur Wheat

1 cup bulgur wheat
1 tablespoon safflower oil
2 cups boiling water

Heat oil and sauté bulgur for 5 minutes, stirring constantly. Add water, cover pot, and lower flame. Cook for 10 minutes. 4 servings.

ALTERNATE METHOD: Place one cup bulgur in 5 cups cold water and let stand 45 minutes. Scoop out and press between palms of your hands to squeeze out excess water. This is a particularly good method for preparing bulgur wheat to be used in salads with fresh fruits or vegetables.

Contains protein, iron, calcium, phosphorus, vitamins A and B.

Cooked Pinto Beans (Frijoles)

1 cup pinto beans
3 to 4 cups water
2 teaspoons honey
2 cloves garlic, minced

2 teaspoons paprika*
1 teaspoon chili powder*
  Sea salt to taste

Wash and sort the beans. Add water and soak overnight in the
refrigerator. Next morning add honey and garlic and bring the
mixture to a boil. Reduce heat, cover and let simmer about 3 or 4
hours, or until the juice has slightly thickened. After the first 2 hours
of cooking, add the paprika and chili powder. Season with salt
during the last half hour of cooking time. 4 servings.

Contains protein, calcium, phosphorus, vitamins A and B.

* Omit these seasonings when you are preparing beans for children under
three years old.

Cooked Chick-peas, Kidney Beans or Adzuki Beans

1 cup chick-peas (or beans)
4 cups water

Soak chick-peas in water for at least 3 to 4 hours before cooking.
Drain chick-peas and add 4 cups water. Bring to a full rolling boil
and cook covered over a low flame for about 2 hours. Remove
cover and cook over a low flame until liquid boils away. 3 to 5
servings.

Contains protein, calcium, phosphorus, vitamins A and B.

Alternate Quick Method for Preparing Beans

(Use this technique for beans that usually require overnight soaking
such as kidney, pinto, or soybeans.)

4 cups water
1 cup beans

Bring water to a full rolling boil and place beans in the water.
Remove from heat and let beans stand in the water until they are
cool. Then reheat and let the beans come to a boil; reduce the heat,
cover, and cook for 2 to 3 hours.

Cooked Couscous

 1 cup couscous
 2 cups boiling water
 1 tablespoon safflower oil

Bring water to a boil and pour in couscous. Add oil and cook for about 2 minutes or until water is almost completely absorbed. Stir occasionally. Remove from heat, cover tightly and let stand for 10 to 12 minutes. Toss well with a fork to insure grains are separate, light, and not sticky. 3 to 4 servings.

Contains protein, iron, calcium, phosphorus, vitamins A and B.

VEGETABLES

Steamed Vegetables

 2 cups vegetables, washed and cut
 1 inch water in bottom of vegetable steamer

Use 1 vegetable or an assortment together in steaming. Slice vegetables such as carrots or green beans on the diagonal into pieces. Cut vegetables such as broccoli and cauliflower into flowerets. Vegetables such as onions are chopped up. Heat water in steamer until a great deal of steam is generated. Put vegetables in steamer tray and into steamer. Cover and steam until done, about 7 to 10 minutes. 2 to 3 servings.

Sautéed Vegetables

 2 cups vegetables, washed and cut
 4 tablespoons vegetable oil
 2 tablespoons Tamari soy sauce

Prepare vegetables as in Steamed Vegetables (above). Heat oil in wok or skillet until very hot. Add vegetables and keep stirring. Make sure all sides are coated with the oil. Add soy sauce after the first 5 minutes of cooking, stirring it in well. Sauté until done, about 7 to 10 minutes. 2 to 3 servings.

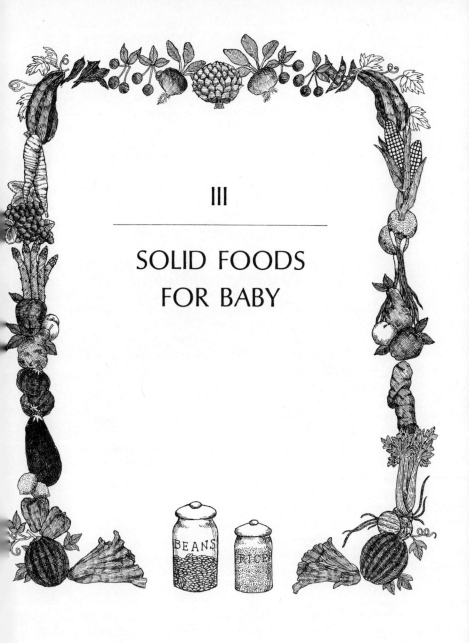

III

SOLID FOODS
FOR BABY

SOYBEANS

Sweet little soybeans, oh so Good for you!
A tiny boy who ate 'em just grew and grew and grew. . . .
—MISS ANN

Soybeans are definitely one of the important foods of the future—when people finally become aware of that little bean that's been around since ancient times. It's infinitely variable; in its many forms it can become sprouts, cheese, curd, milk, flour, bean pulp or a meatlike pulp. It's a vitally important source of protein, essential amino acids, and practically all known vitamins.

It's the cornerstone of a vegetarian diet.

Simple Soybean Pulp

1 cup Cooked Soybeans (page 41)
Splash of milk

Combine soybeans and milk in blender and purée until soybeans are completely dissolved into a thick, pulpy paste. Use more milk for a smoother texture. 4 servings.

Serve from 6 months on. It's good to keep this on hand at all times. Make this the main course, along with some fruit and a vegetable, or give the baby a couple of tablespoonfuls with his major meal. It's important to emphasize soybeans if you are raising a vegetarian child.

Contains protein, iron, phosphorus, calcium, vitamins A and B.

Soybean-Cheese Meal

½ cup Simple Soybean Pulp (above)
2 tablespoons grated mild Cheddar cheese
2 teaspoons Tamari soy sauce

Combine all ingredients in blender and purée to the consistency of mashed potatoes. 1 or 2 servings.

Serve from 6 months on. Use this frequently as part of baby's dinner meal.

Contains protein, iron, phosphorus, calcium, vitamins A and B.

Soy Pancakes (Best Breakfast)

⅔ cup Cooked Soybeans (page 41)
1 egg
⅓ teaspoon cinnamon
   Splash of milk

In a blender combine the egg with soybeans and purée to a smooth paste. Add cinnamon and stir in enough milk to make a creamy, slightly heavy, but not runny, batter. Grease a skillet or griddle lightly with oil and heat to the point where a drop of water will crackle and sizzle in the skillet. Pour in the batter to make 2 medium-sized pancakes. Turn the heat down and brown the pancakes slowly on both sides. Serve with soybean oleomargarine and honey. Makes 1 serving.

Serve from 6 months on; just mash slightly for a baby with no teeth. This is a wonderful breakfast food because it is incredibly rich in protein and vitamins. Children love it because it seems like a sweet treat. My son seemed to prefer these pancakes to any other breakfast food and I often served it 3 or 4 times a week. I heartily recommend it.

Contains protein, calcium, iron, lecithin, phosphorus, vitamins A and B.

A Recipe of Many Variations

½ cup steamed green beans or broccoli (page 46 for Steamed
      Vegetables)
 2 tablespoons ground sunflower seeds
 1 heaping tablespoon yogurt
½ cup Simple Soybean Pulp (page 51)
¼ cup Cooked Bulgur Wheat (page 44) or Cooked Couscous
      (page 46)
¼ cup Steamed Brown Rice (page 42)
      Tamari soy sauce to taste

Chop up green beans or broccoli well and combine with sunflower
seeds and yogurt in blender. Purée to a smooth paste. Add soybean
pulp, bulgur wheat, and rice and purée until well mixed. Season to
taste with Tamari soy sauce. As your child gets more teeth, you can
blend this dinner to a coarser consistency or use cooked soybeans
(page 41) instead of pulp. 2 servings.

Serve from 6 months on. This meal lends itself to many variations,
both mine and yours. Use it as a basis for building many nourishing
meals.

Contains protein, iron, calcium, lecithin, phosphorus, vitamins
A, B, C, D and E.

Bean-Bean Dinner

 2 tablespoons safflower oil
½ cup fresh green beans
 2 tablespoons pine nuts
 2 teaspoons Tamari soy sauce
      Splash of tomato juice
½ cup Simple Soybean Pulp (page 51)

Heat oil in skillet and add green beans. Sauté until beans are
thoroughly cooked, about 15 to 20 minutes. Add pine nuts and continue to sauté until nuts are browned. Add soy sauce and sauté for

about 3 more minutes. Put green beans and nuts in blender with enough tomato juice to facilitate puréeing. Purée to a thick paste. Add soybean pulp and stir well. 2 servings.

VARIATION: Use carrots instead of green beans.

Contains protein, iron, phosphorus, calcium, vitamins A and B.

Max's New Mexican Treat

½ cup Simple Soybean Pulp (page 51)
½ cup pine nuts, ground
   Dash of yogurt
   Tamari soy sauce to taste

Mix together the soybean pulp and pine nuts. Add enough yogurt to achieve a custardlike consistency. Season with Tamari soy sauce to taste. 2 servings.
Serve from 6 months. Good for dinner.

Contains protein, calcium, iron, phosphorus, lecithin, vitamins A, B and C.

Baby's Bounty

½ cup Simple Soybean Pulp (page 51)
½ cup Basic Baked Squash (page 73)
¼ cup stewed tomatoes
 2 tablespoons grated Cheddar cheese

Combine all ingredients in blender and stir together well. Serve warm. 2 servings.
Serve from 6 months on. This makes a good first food for babies.

Contains protein, iron, phosphorus, calcium, vitamins A, B and C.

Good and Hearty Baby Dinner

   2 tablespoons corn oil
⅓ of a Spanish onion, chopped
   2 tablespoons water
   2 teaspoons Tamari soy sauce
½ cup Simple Soybean Pulp (page 51)
½ cup Cooked Lentils (page 43)
⅓ cup stewed tomatoes

Heat oil in skillet and add onions. Sauté slowly over medium heat until onions are slightly brown and wilted, about 15 to 20 minutes. Add water and Tamari soy sauce during last 5 minutes of cooking. Pour into blender and add remaining ingredients. Purée to the consistency of a heavy pudding. 2 servings.

Serve from 6 months on. Serve this dinner frequently to a vegetarian baby.

Contains protein, calcium, phosphorus, iron, vitamins A, B and C.

GRAINS AND DRIED BEANS

Winter Night Casserole

   1 small zucchini squash (raw)
   1 small ripe tomato
⅔ cup cottage cheese
⅛ cup milk
   1 egg yolk (optional)
   1 cup Steamed Brown Rice (page 42)
   2 teaspoons grated Monterey jack cheese
      Sesame-sea salt

Chop up zucchini and tomato and combine with cottage cheese, milk and egg (if used). Purée in blender until smooth pastelike consistency is developed. Mix batter with brown rice (of a mushy consistency, if child has few teeth). Sprinkle with grated cheese and sesame-sea salt. Place under broiler for a few seconds, until cheese melts. Serve warm. 1 or 2 servings.

Serve from 6 months on.

Contains protein, calcium, phosphorus, potassium, sodium, vitamins A, B$_{12}$, niacin and C.

Tijuana Lunchtime for Baby

½ green pepper
½ Spanish onion
     Safflower oil
 1 beaten egg
⅔ cup Steamed Brown Rice (page 42)
 2 tablespoons grated Cheddar cheese
 1 tablespoon Tamari soy sauce

Chop pepper and onion finely and sauté in safflower oil over low heat until wilted and softened, about 30 to 40 minutes. Set aside. Mix egg with rice, cheese, and soy sauce and add pepper and onion. Bake at 350° for 20 to 30 minutes. Serve warm. 1 or 2 servings.

Serve from 6 months on, using rice of a mushy consistency if served to younger baby or one with few teeth. Serve to older children using rice of a more sharply defined grain and large chunks of pepper and onion.

Contains protein, calcium, lecithin, phosphorus, potassium, sodium, vitamins A, B, niacin and C.

Rice and Vegetables

½ cup Steamed Brown Rice (page 42)
⅓ cup Hijiki Sea Vegetable (page 142)
⅓ cup Brussels Sprouts, Steamed (page 46)

2 tablespoons ground sunflower seeds
Dash of yogurt
Tamari soy sauce to taste

Combine rice, hijiki, sprouts and seeds in blender; purée until completely dissolved. Moisten with a dash of yogurt and season with Tamari soy sauce to taste. 1 or 2 servings.
Serve from 8 months on.

Contains protein, calcium, phosphorus, iron, vitamins A, C and D.

Seafood Fare

½ cup carrots, chopped
½ cup Mushy Rice for Baby (page 42)
⅓ cup Hijiki Sea Vegetable (page 142)

Steam carrots in a vegetable steamer until thoroughly cooked and softened, about 15 to 20 minutes. Combine in blender with rice and hijiki and purée to a smooth consistency. 2 servings.
Serve from 6 months on. Seaweed is definitely a food of the future and an excellent vegetable for the vegetarian child.

Contains protein, phosphorus, iron, calcium, vitamins A and C.

VARIATION: Use other vegetables in place of the carrots such as green beans, broccoli or squash. Or use Simple Soybean Pulp (page 51) in place of the brown rice.

Luscious Lentils and Rice

½ Spanish onion
Safflower oil
Water
1 tablespoon blackstrap molasses
2 teaspoons Tamari soy sauce
⅔ cup Cooked Lentils and Rice (page 57)

Chop onion and sauté slowly in oil until wilted and browned, about 20 minutes. Add a bit of water now and then to keep it moist.

Stir in molasses and soy sauce when you remove onion from the fire. Combine with rice and lentils in blender and purée to the consistency of oatmeal. 2 servings.

Serve from 6 months on. This is an excellent dinner and should be served frequently.

Contains protein, calcium, iron, phosphorus, potassium, sodium, and vitamin C.

An Armenian Dinner Deluxe

    4 tablespoons yogurt
    4 heaping tablespoons Cooked Lentils (page 43)
    2 tablespoons peanut butter
    1 teaspoon molasses

Combine all ingredients in blender and purée to the texture of a heavy oatmeal. 1 serving.

Serve from 6 months on. This is a good dinner dish.

Contains protein, calcium, iron, phosphorus, potassium, sodium, vitamins A, B and niacin.

Wheatie Breakfast

    4 black mission figs
      Apple juice to cover
    ⅓ cup yogurt
    ½ cup Cooked Bulgur Wheat (page 44)

Soak figs overnight in apple juice. Put in blender with apple juice and yogurt and purée until milk shake consistency is reached, adding a bit more apple juice if necessary. Mix with bulgur wheat and serve. 1 to 2 servings.

Serve from 6 months on. This can also be served as a breakfast food to the whole family.

Contains protein, calcium, iron, phosphorus, potassium, vitamins A, B and niacin.

Provincetown Snack

½ cup dried apricots
½ apple
½ pear
1 teaspoon honey
⅓ cup yogurt
½ cup Cooked Bulgur Wheat (page 44)

Soak apricots overnight in water to soften; core apple and chop; chop pear; combine fruit with soaking water, honey and yogurt in blender. Purée to a puddinglike texture and fold in bulgur. For a toothless baby, purée the bulgur until completely dissolved into the fruit purée. 2 servings.

Serve from 6 months on. This makes a good breakfast for the entire family.

Contains phosphorus, potassium, sodium, vitamins A and C, niacin, also protein, calcium and vitamin B.

Blue Bulgur Lunch

½ cup fresh blueberries
⅓ cup yogurt
1½ teaspoons apricot concentrate
1 teaspoon honey
½ cup Cooked Bulgur Wheat (page 44)

Combine blueberries, yogurt, apricot concentrate and honey. Purée in blender until puddinglike texture is reached. Fold in Bulgur. 2 servings.

Serve from 8 months on. Purée the bulgur with the fruit purée if baby has not learned to chew at all.

Contains protein, calcium, potassium, vitamins A, B and C.

Halloween Lunch

⅓ of a small pumpkin
2 tablespoons ricotta cheese
2 tablespoons yogurt
1 teaspoon honey
   Splash of apricot nectar
⅓ cup Cooked Bulgur Wheat (page 44)

Remove seeds, stringy portion and outside shell of pumpkin. Cut into small pieces and cover with boiling water. Cook until tender, about 20 to 25 minutes. Drain and combine in blender with cheese, yogurt, honey and nectar. Purée to a soft-pudding texture, using more nectar if necessary. Fold in bulgur. 2 or 3 servings.
Serve from 8 months on.

Contains protein, calcium, phosphorus, potassium, vitamins A and C.

Arabian Lunch

1 ripe peach
3 tablespoons yogurt
1 tablespoon tahini
½ cup Cooked Couscous (page 46)

Combine peach, yogurt and tahini in blender; purée to a smooth, even consistency. Fold in couscous. 1 or 2 servings.
Serve from 8 months on; for a baby with no teeth, purée couscous in blender with other ingredients.

Contains protein, calcium, vitamins A, B, C and E.

Tangerian Treat

1 teaspoon blackstrap molasses
½ cup cooked mashed carrots
   Splash of apple juice
½ cup Cooked Couscous (page 46)

Mix molasses into carrots. Use a bit of apple juice to achieve a puddinglike texture. Stir in couscous and blend. 1 or 2 servings.
Serve from 8 months on.

Contains iron, potassium, sodium, vitamins A, B and C.

Chick-peas Alexandria

½ cup Cooked Chick-peas (page 45)
2 tablespoons tahini
1 tablespoon ricotta cheese
½ teaspoon lemon juice
2 tablespoons yogurt

Combine all ingredients in blender and purée to a puddinglike consistency. 1 or 2 servings.
Serve from 6 months on. This is a good evening meal.

Contains protein, calcium, phosphorus, vitamins A, B and C.

Chick-pea Chow

½ cup Cooked Chick-peas (page 45)
5 heaping tablespoons yogurt
2 heaping teaspoons finely minced parsley
¾ teaspoon Tamari soy sauce
   Sesame-sea salt

When cooking chick-peas, save the last few spoonfuls of cooking water. Place chick-peas, cooking water, and 3 tablespoons yogurt in blender and purée until chick-peas are broken down and slightly mashed. Add parsley, soy sauce and remaining yogurt; purée until an oatmeallike consistency is reached. Serve sprinkled lightly with sesame-sea salt. 2 servings.
Serve from 8 months on. This makes an excellent dinner any time.

Contains protein, calcium, phosphorus, potassium, vitamins A and B.

Moroccan Dinner

>   ½ cup carrots, sliced about ½ inch thick
>   ½ cup Cooked Chick-peas (page 45)
>   ¾ teaspoon Tamari soy sauce
>   1 heaping teaspoon blackstrap molasses
>   ¼ cup Cooked Couscous (page 46)

Steam carrots in vegetable steamer until very soft and easy to mash. Let cool and reserve the steaming water. Put carrots in blender with enough steaming water to purée to a custardlike consistency. Add chick-peas and more carrot water. Purée to an oatmeallike consistency. Add soy sauce and molasses. Fold in couscous and serve. 1 or 2 servings.

Serve from 8 months on. This makes a good winter dinner.

Contains protein, iron, phosphorus, potassium, niacin, vitamins A and C.

Millet-Broccoli Dinner

>   ½ cup broccoli, cut into small pieces
>   1 teaspoon lemon juice
>   1 teaspoon Tamari soy sauce
>   2 heaping tablespoons yogurt
>   ½ cup Cooked Millet (page 44)

Steam broccoli in vegetable steamer until very tender, about 15 minutes. Combine in blender with lemon juice, soy sauce, and yogurt. Purée to an oatmeallike texture and fold into millet. 1 or 2 servings.

Serve from 8 months on. To serve a baby with no teeth, you may want to run mixture, including millet, through the blender again.

Contains protein, calcium, iron, phosphorus, potassium, niacin, vitamins A, B and C.

Maxie's Millet Surprise

　　Safflower or corn oil for sautéing
⅓　of a large Spanish onion, finely chopped
　　Water
½　ripe tomato, finely chopped
¾　teaspoon Tamari soy sauce
　　Sesame-sea salt
⅓　cup cooked millet (page 44)

Heat oil and sauté onion, stirring occasionally, until completely wilted, about 30 minutes. Add water occasionally to keep onion slightly moist. Add tomato and soy sauce and simmer for 4 or 5 minutes. Let cool and pour mixture into blender and chop coarsely for a few seconds. Mix with millet and sprinkle with sesame-sea salt. 1 or 2 servings.
　　Serve from 8 months on. This dish makes a good dinner.

Contains potassium, vitamins A and C.

EGGS

> Higgelty, piggelty, my black hen,
> She lays eggs for gentlemen.
> —MOTHER GOOSE

Very Easy Breakfast

　1　soft-boiled egg
　1　toasted slice whole-grain bread

Crumble toast into bite-sized pieces and put egg on top; mix together until toast is softened. 1 serving.
　　Serve from 4 to 6 months on.

Contains protein, iron, calcium, phosphorus, potassium, sodium, vitamins A and B.

Lentil-Egg Breakfast

    Safflower oil
1 egg
⅓ cup Cooked Lentils (page 43)
2 teaspoons grated Cheddar cheese

Heat oil in skillet and beat up the egg; add egg to oil and begin to scramble. When about halfway finished, add lentils and cheese and finish scrambling. 1 serving.

Serve from 8 months on. This is actually a fine way to serve eggs to the whole family.

Contains protein, calcium, phosphorus, potassium, sodium, and vitamin A.

NOTE: There are more egg recipes for baby in Chapter V, with larger servings for the whole family.

FRUITS

First Meal

½ a ripe banana
1 tablespoon yogurt
1 heaping teaspoon Basic Cereal for Baby (page 34)

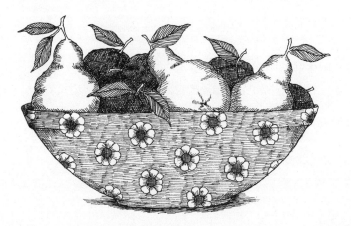

Combine all ingredients in blender and purée to a custardlike texture. 1 serving.

Serve from 3 months on.

Contains protein, calcium, phosphorus, potassium, vitamins A, B and C.

Winter Breakfast Pudding

    6 to 8 dried apricots
        Apple juice to cover
    ⅔ cup yogurt

Soak apricots overnight in apple juice until completely softened; place juice and apricots in blender and purée until dissolved into a smooth paste. Add yogurt and stir in. 2 servings.

Serve from 3 months on. Also serve this to the whole family as a dessert. Sprinkle some chopped walnuts on top for a treat.

Contains protein, calcium, phosphorus, potassium, sodium, vitamins A and B.

Cooked Cranberries

    1 pound fresh cranberries, washed and sorted
    1½ cups apple juice
    ¾ cup honey
    2 teaspoons grated orange rind
        Freshly grated nutmeg

Combine all ingredients in saucepan and bring to boil; reduce heat and let simmer until berries begin to pop, about 5 minutes. Remove from heat and cover. Let stand until lukewarm and then refrigerate. 4 to 6 servings.

Serve from 4 to 6 months on. Cooked cranberries are very good to have around. Because of their liquid consistency, they combine well with other fruits and vegetables when making puréed baby food. They also make a good ingredient for blended drinks.

Contains potassium, calcium, vitamins A and C.

Cape Cod Breakfast

½ cup Cooked Cranberries (above)
½ cup Abby Van Derek's Incredible Granola (page 32)
½ orange, peeled and divided into segments

Combine all ingredients in blender and purée to a puddinglike texture. 1 or 2 servings.
Serve from 6 months on.

Contains protein, calcium, phosphorus, potassium, sodium, niacin, vitamins A, B, C, D and E.

Date Delight

4 pitted dates
½ a baked acorn squash (page 73)
½ a ripe papaya
1 heaping teaspoon brewer's yeast
½ teaspoon honey

Combine all ingredients in blender and purée to a puddinglike consistency. 1 serving.
Serve from 6 months on. A good lunch or dinner.

Contains protein, iron, calcium, phosphorus, potassium, sodium, vitamins A, B, niacin and C.

Fancy Breakfast

½ cup chopped pineapple, cooked or fresh
½ cup yogurt
¼ cup wheat germ

Combine all ingredients in blender and purée to chunky consistency. 2 or 3 servings.

Serve from 6 months on for breakfast; serve to older children as is or pour over whole-grain cereal and add milk.

Contains protein, calcium, iron, phosphorus, potassium, vitamins A, B, niacin, C and E.

Pears Perchance

    3 dried pear halves or 1 fresh pear
      Apple juice to cover
    ½ cup yogurt
    ⅛ teaspoon powdered ginger
    2 heaping teaspoons ground nuts or sunflower seeds

Soak pears overnight in apple juice; place in blender and purée until liquefied. Stir in remaining ingredients. 1 or 2 servings.
Serve from 4 to 6 months on. Makes a good meal anytime.

Contains calcium, phosphorus, potassium, protein and vitamin D.

Plum Nutty

    2 ripe plums
    4 tablespoons cottage cheese
    2 tablespoons yogurt
    1 heaping tablespoon peanut butter
    1 teaspoon honey

Chop plums coarsely and combine with remaining ingredients in blender. Purée until a puddinglike consistency is developed. 2 servings.
Serve from 6 months on for a quick lunch or dinner.

Contains protein, calcium, phosphorus, potassium, vitamins A, B and C.

Pumpkin Pudding

⅓ a small pumpkin
1 egg yolk
1 teaspoon ginger
1 tablespoon cream cheese
4 tablespoons yogurt
1 teaspoon honey
   Splash of peach nectar

Remove seeds, stringy portion, and outside shell of pumpkin. Cut into small pieces and cover with boiling water. Cook until tender, about 20 to 25 minutes. Drain and combine with remaining ingredients in blender. Purée to a custardlike consistency. 2 servings. Serve from 8 months on.

Contains protein, calcium, vitamin A and lecithin.

Afternoon Avocados

½ ripe avocado
½ ripe banana
¼ cup cottage cheese
   Splash of apple juice

Peel and chop avocado and banana; combine in blender with remaining ingredients and purée to a custardlike texture. 1 or 2 servings. Serve from 6 months on. Use this for lunch or dinner.

Contains protein, calcium. phosphorus, potassium, sodium, vitamins A, B, niacin, C and lecithin.

East End Lunch

1 ripe banana
1 tablespoon tahini

    1 tablespoon almond butter
⅓ cup Mushy Rice (page 42)
    Splash of orange juice

Combine all ingredients in blender and purée to a rich, thick
oatmeallike texture, using a bit or orange juice to keep it moist. 1 or
2 servings.
Serve from 8 months on.

Contains protein, vitamins A, B and E.

> Up in the green orchard there is a green tree
> The finest of pippins that ever you see;
> The apples are ripe, and ready to fall,
> And Reuben and Robin shall gather them all.
> —MOTHER GOOSE

Apple Supreme

½ apple, cored and cut into small pieces
½ butternut squash, baked (page 73)
 4 tablespoons yogurt
 4 tablespoons ricotta cheese
 2 teaspoons honey

Combine all ingredients in blender and purée to a smooth,
custardlike consistency. 2 servings.
Serve from 6 months on. This makes a good dinner.

Contains protein, calcium, potassium, vitamins A, B and C.

Fruity Breakfast or Lunch

½ ripe mango
10 pitted bing cherries
10 fresh strawberries
½ cup yogurt
    Brown rice or cereal

Scoop out mango and combine with cherries, strawberries and yogurt in blender. Purée to milkshake consistency. Pour over steamed rice or cereal. 1 or 2 servings.

Serve from 6 months on, using mushy rice if served to younger baby or one with few teeth.

VARIATION: Serve to older children as rice pudding by combining fruit purée, rice, raisins softened in juice, and walnut pieces.

Contains protein, calcium, phosphorus, potassium, vitamins A, B, C and E.

8 A.M. *Oranges*

6 dried apricot halves
  Orange juice
1 orange
4 tablespoons Abby Van Derek's Incredible Granola (page 32)
2 tablespoons sunflower seeds
2 tablespoons honey

Soak apricots overnight in orange juice; peel orange and separate into segments. Combine apricots, juice and orange segments in blender and purée until completely dissolved. Add remaining ingredients and purée again, using more orange juice to moisten mixture, if necessary. 1 or 2 servings.

Serve from 6 months on. Good for breakfast.

Contains protein, calcium, phosphorus, potassium, sodium, niacin, vitamins A, B, C and D.

Milanese Morning Custard

3 dried peach halves or 1 fresh peach
  Peach nectar to cover
2 tablespoons ricotta cheese
2 tablespoons yogurt

Soak dried peaches overnight in nectar. Pour nectar and peaches into blender and purée to heavy puddinglike consistency. Add cheese and yogurt and purée again. 2 servings.

Serve from 6 months on. This is a really delicious, cheesecake-tasting breakfast or lunch dish.

Contains protein, calcium, phosphorus, sodium, vitamins A, B and C.

Funny Dinner

    1 small ripe peach
    4 heaping tablespoons cottage cheese
    1 heaping tablespoon peanut butter
    1 ripe banana

Chop fruit and combine with remaining ingredients in blender. Purée until of smooth-paste consistency.

Serve from 4 to 6 months on as lunch or dinner.

Contains protein, calcium, phosphorus, potassium, sodium, vitamins A, B, niacin and C.

Prune Pudding

    3 dried prunes
      Cherry juice to cover
    1 apple
    ½ cup yogurt
    2 heaping teaspoons ground nuts (filberts or hazelnuts)

Soak prunes overnight in cherry juice; place in blender and purée to a puddinglike consistency. Core apple, but leave unpeeled, and chop into small pieces. Add apple and remaining ingredients to blender and purée to a custardlike texture. 2 servings.

Serve from 6 months on. Good anytime.

Contains protein, calcium, phosphorus, potassium and vitamins A and B.

Prunes à la Roma

    3 stewed prunes, pitted
    ½ a ripe banana
    3 tablespoons ricotta cheese
    3 tablespoons yogurt
       Splash of prune juice

Combine all ingredients in blender and purée to a custardlike texture. 1 or 2 servings.

Serve from 8 months on. This makes a good breakfast for a constipated baby.

Contains protein, calcium, potassium, phosphorus, vitamins A, B and C.

Figs à la Barrow Street
(a Christmastime breakfast)

    4 to 6 dried black mission figs
       Cherry juice to cover
    1 cup yogurt
    ¼ cup cottage cheese
    1 teaspoon honey (optional)

Soften figs overnight in refrigerator in a liberal amount of cherry juice. Pour juice and figs into blender and purée until smooth puddinglike texture is achieved. Add remaining ingredients and purée again. 2 to 3 servings.

Serve from 4 to 6 months on; also serve as a pudding dessert to the whole family. Some sources (unproven) say black mission figs help to prevent baldness, so serve this to scanty-topped males.

Contains protein, calcium, iron, phosphorus, potassium, sodium, vitamins A, B and C.

Miss Ann's Raisin Yogurt

>   2 cups goat's-milk Yogurt (page 31)
>   Vanilla bean
> ⅓ cup raisins
>   Apple juice to cover
>   1 teaspoon honey (optional)

Prepare yogurt in usual manner with fresh goat's milk; drop in a vanilla bean while mixture is fermenting. Soften raisins overnight in refrigerator in liberal amount of apple juice. Pour juice, raisins and honey into blender and purée until milkshake consistency is developed. Stir in yogurt and serve. 3 to 4 servings.

Serve from 4 to 6 months on. This dish is also a good snack for nursing mothers and pregnant women.

Contains protein, calcium, phosphorus, potassium, vitamins A, B and C.

VEGETABLES

Basic Baked Squash
(for butternut or acorn squash)

>   1 squash
>   1 tablespoon vegetable oil
>   1 teaspoon tupelo honey
>   1 teaspoon butter, optional

Preheat oven to 350° F. Cut squash in half and rub flesh side of each half with vegetable oil and then honey. Sprinkle lightly with cinnamon, nutmeg, ground cloves, or a combination. Bake for about 1 hour and 10 minutes, or until flesh is very soft. Mash with butter, if desired. 2 or 3 servings.

Serve from 6 months on. This is a very good first vegetable to introduce. Its soft and pulpy texture, along with bananas, makes it easy to serve to a new baby.

Contains calcium, phosphorus, vitamins A and C.

Butternut Squash à la Malicia

    1 orange
    ½ cup baked butternut squash (page 73)
    ½ cup cereal (see Chapter II)
    1 teaspoon honey
    2 tablespoons yogurt
      Splash of orange juice

Peel orange and divide into segments. Combine in blender with remaining ingredients and purée to the consistency of oatmeal. 1 or 2 servings.

Serve from 6 months on.

Contains protein, calcium, phosphorus, potassium, sodium, niacin, vitamins A, B, C and E.

Autumn Lunch

    1 medium butternut squash, baked (page 73)
      Pinch of nutmeg
      Pinch of cinnamon
    1 teaspoon honey (optional)
    1 cup yogurt

Spoon out baked squash into blender; combine with remaining ingredients and purée to the consistency of mashed potatoes. 2 servings.

Serve from 4 to 6 months on. Use as dinner vegetable for older children.

Contains protein, calcium, phosphorus, potassium, sodium, vitamins A, B, C and lecithin.

A Dinner Divine

    1 acorn squash, baked (page 73)
      Pinch of freshly grated nutmeg

1 ripe banana
1 egg yolk
    Splash of apple juice

Put squash in blender with remaining ingredients. Purée until puddinglike consistency is reached. 2 servings.

Serve from 4 to 6 months on as a dinner meal, or serve to older children as a pudding treat.

Contains protein, calcium, lecithin, phosphorus, potassium, vitamins A and C.

Squashberry Snack

¾ cup baked acorn squash (page 73)
½ cup Cooked Cranberries (page 65)
1 teaspoon brewer's yeast

Combine all ingredients in blender and purée to a custardlike texture. 1 or 2 servings.

Serve from 6 months on.

Contains protein, calcium, phosphorus, potassium, iron, niacin, sodium, vitamins A, B, C and lecithin.

Squash Lunch

2 medium-size yellow summer squash
1 ripe banana
¾ cup yogurt

Chop squash and banana; liquefy in blender with yogurt. 1 or 2 servings.

Serve from 4 to 6 months on.

Contains protein, calcium, phosphorus, potassium, vitamins A, B and C.

Indian Breakfast Treat

   1 medium yellow summer squash (raw)
   1 small ripe peach (raw)
  ⅔ cup yogurt
   1 teaspoon honey (optional)

Coarsely chop squash and peach; combine with yogurt and honey in blender. Purée until ingredients have been reduced to very small particles. 1 or 2 servings.

Serve from 6 to 8 months on. Serve as is or combined with whole grain cereal and milk for breakfast.

Contains protein, calcium, phosphorus, potassium, sodium, vitamins A, B and C.

Blue Plate Special

   1 medium yellow summer squash
  ⅓ cup Cooked Bulgur Wheat (page 44)
  ¾ cup yogurt
   1 teaspoon honey
  ¼ cup apple juice or tomato juice

Chop squash and combine with remaining ingredients in blender and purée until a milkshake-like, or slightly thicker, consistency is reached. 1 or 2 servings.

Serve from 4 to 6 months on. This makes a good dinner.

Contains protein, iron, calcium, phosphorus, potassium, niacin, vitamins A, B, and C.

Wednesday Night Dinner

   1 small yellow summer squash
  ½ cup cottage cheese
  2 tablespoons milk

3 heaping tablespoons Mushy Rice (page 42)
Sesame-sea salt

Chop squash and combine with cheese and milk in blender; purée until rich pudding consistency is reached. Remove from blender and stir in brown rice. Sprinkle with sesame-sea salt. 1 or 2 servings.
Serve from 6 months on.

Contains protein, calcium, phosphorus, potassium, sodium, vitamins A, B, C, E, niacin and lecithin.

Sunday's Squash

    1 small yellow summer squash
    1 tablespoon peanut butter
    1 teaspoon honey
    ½ cup cottage cheese
      Splash of tomato juice

Chop squash coarsely and combine with remaining ingredients in blender. Purée to a puddinglike consistency. 1 or 2 servings.
Serve from 6 months on. Good high protein dinner.

Contains protein, calcium, phosphorus, potassium, sodium, vitamins A, B, niacin and C.

Baby's Gazpacho

    1 medium zucchini squash, raw
    1 ripe tomato
    ⅔ cup cottage cheese
    ½ cup yogurt
    5 tablespoons milk
      Sesame-sea salt to taste

Chop up zucchini and tomato and steam together for 7 to 10 minutes. Pour into blender. Add remaining ingredients and purée to a rich, slightly heavy consistency. 2 servings.
Serve from 6 months on.

Contains protein, calcium, phosphorus, potassium, sodium, vitamins A, B and C.

Turkish Tomato Salad

    1 medium-size ripe tomato, chopped
    1 medium-size yellow summer squash, chopped
   ¼ cup celery, finely chopped
    5 heaping tablespoons yogurt
    2 teaspoons ground nuts (peanuts or cashews)
   ½ teaspoon fresh dill, finely chopped

Combine all ingredients in blender and purée until a heavy oatmeallike consistency is reached. 2 servings.

Serve from 8 months on. Good for a lunch or dinner salad.

VARIATION: When baby has 8 to 10 teeth and can chew well, stir in 2 tablespoons of cooked brown rice just before serving.

Contains protein, calcium, phosphorus, potassium, and vitamins A, B and C.

Miss Ann's Tomato Surprise

    Safflower oil
    2 yellow summer squash, sliced thinly on the diagonal and halved
   ¼ cup finely chopped Spanish onion
    Pinch of basil
   ¼ cup diced Muenster cheese
   ½ cup diced fresh tomatoes
   ½ teaspoon sea salt
   ½ teaspoon buckwheat honey

Heat oil in skillet and add squash, onion and basil. Sauté a few minutes, stirring constantly. Cover skillet and let simmer 10 minutes. Add cheese and stir well. Remove from heat. In the same skillet that squash was cooked in, add tomatoes, salt, and honey. Sauté 4 to 5 minutes. Add tomatoes to squash and put in blender. Purée to an oatmeallike texture. 2 servings.

Serve from 8 months on.

Contains calcium, phosphorus, potassium, sodium, niacin, vitamins A, B, C, E and lecithin.

Baby's Mexican Dinner

½ ripe avocado
½ medium ripe tomato
⅔ cup cottage cheese
4 tablespoons yogurt
1 teaspoon lemon juice

Peel avocado and combine with remaining ingredients in blender; purée until chunky oatmeallike consistency is developed. Serve immediately. 2 servings.

Serve from 8 months on. When baby has some teeth, add a piece of toasted whole-grain bread spread with sesame or apple butter.

Contains protein, calcium, phosphorus, potassium, sodium, vitamins A, B and C.

Eggplant Elegante

Safflower oil
½ cup eggplant, peeled and diced
⅓ cup tomato, diced
3 tablespoons ricotta cheese
Splash of tomato juice

Heat oil in skillet and sauté eggplant for about 5 minutes; add tomato and cook together for another 3 to 5 minutes. Combine in blender with cheese. Use a bit of tomato juice to moisten, if necessary. Purée to a puddinglike consistency. 1 or 2 servings.

Serve from 8 months on. This makes a good dinner.

Contains protein, calcium, lecithin, potassium, vitamins A, B, C and E.

Basic Baked Yams or Sweet Potatoes

> 1 yam or sweet potato
>   Vegetable oil

Preheat oven to 350° F. Scrub yam thoroughly with a vegetable brush, using a very mild castile soap solution. Rinse thoroughly and dry. Rub surface of yam with vegetable oil and place in oven. Cook for about 1 hour and 15 minutes, or until pulp is very soft. Prepared this way, the skins are edible and nutritious. Serves 1 or 2.

Serve from 4 months on.

Contains protein, calcium, phosphorus, vitamins A and C.

Yam Pone Poke

> ½ sweet potato, baked
> 1 tablespoon corn oil
> 1 apple
> 1 ripe banana
> 1 teaspoon honey
> ¼ cup wheat germ

Mash sweet potato with corn oil until light and fluffy. Remove core from apple, but do not peel. Chop apple into pieces and combine with banana chunks and honey in blender. Purée until a puddinglike texture is reached. Combine with potato and wheat germ. 2 servings.

Serve from 4 months on. Good for a winter dinner.

Contains lecithin, potassium, vitamins A, B, C and E.

Yammy Do

> 3 heaping tablespoons Basic Baked Yam (page 80)
> 2 black mission figs
> 3 heaping tablespoons Cooked Bulgur Wheat (page 44)

⅓ a ripe banana
1 teaspoon honey
   Splash of soy milk

Combine all ingredients in blender with enough soy milk to
purée to the consistency of heavy custard. 2 servings.
Serve from 8 months on. Very good for a winter lunch or dinner.

Contains protein, calcium, iron, phosphorus, potassium, vitamins
A, B, niacin, C and lecithin.

Sweet Potato-Apricot Soufflé

5 dried apricots
   Apricot nectar
½ cup yogurt
½ a medium-size sweet potato, baked (page 80)
1 teaspoon blackstrap molasses

Soak apricots overnight in apricot nectar to cover. Pour apricots
and excess nectar into blender; add yogurt and purée until apricots
are completely dissolved. Add sweet potato and molasses and purée
until a rich, puddinglike texture is reached. Use a bit more apricot
nectar if a lighter texture is desired. 2 servings.
Serve from 4 to 6 months on. This dish makes a good lunch or
dinner in the winter.

Contains protein, calcium, iron, phosphorus, potassium, vitamins
A and C.

Thanksgiving Dinner

½ medium-size sweet potato, baked (page 80)
¼ cup Cooked Bulgur Wheat (page 44)
½ cup yogurt
¼ cup Cooked Cranberries (page 65)
½ teaspoon cinnamon
1 teaspoon honey

Put sweet potato in blender with remaining ingredients and purée to a puddinglike consistency. 1 or 2 servings.

Serve from 4 to 6 months on. This makes a good dinner.

Contains protein, iron, calcium, phosphorus, potassium, vitamins A, B, niacin and C.

Yummy Yams

    1 small tangerine
    ½ baked yam (page 80)
    2 tablespoons yogurt
    1 teaspoon honey
    ¼ teaspoon cinnamon

Peel tangerine and divide into sections; place in blender with remaining ingredients and purée until a custardlike consistency is achieved. 1 or 2 servings.

Serve from 6 months on.

Contains protein, calcium, potassium, vitamins A and C.

Carrotberry Concoction

    1 large fresh carrot, grated
    2 tablespoons yogurt
    3 tablespoons Cooked Cranberries (page 65)
    ½ a ripe banana

Combine all ingredients in blender and purée to the texture of a light pudding. 1 or 2 servings.

Serve from 6 months on. A good light lunch dish.

Contains protein, iron, calcium, phosphorus, potassium, sodium, vitamins A, B and C.

Lunchtime Dish

2 teaspoons raisins
  Splash of apple juice
1 apple, unpeeled
1 large fresh carrot, grated
2 tablespoons yogurt

Soak raisins overnight in apple juice in refrigerator; core apple and chop into small pieces. Combine all ingredients in blender and purée to the consistency of pudding. 1 or 2 servings.
Serve from 6 months on. A good lunch.

Contains protein, iron, calcium, potassium, phosphorus, vitamins A and C.

Baby's Turnip and Carrot Dinner

1 medium carrot, sliced into 1-inch pieces
1 medium turnip, peeled and sliced into bite-sized pieces
  Water
2 tablespoons yogurt
½ teaspoon soybean oleomargarine, melted
½ teaspoon Tamari soy sauce

Simmer carrot and turnip together in small amount of water until tender, about 25 minutes. Drain off cooking water and reserve. Put turnip and carrot in blender and add enough cooking water to moisten. Purée until the texture of mashed potatoes is reached, using more water if necessary. Remove from blender and stir in remaining ingredients. Serve warm, reheating if necessary. 1 or 2 servings.
Serve from 6 months on. This makes a good winter vegetable with a soybean entrée.

Contains protein, calcium, phosphorus, potassium, vitamins A, B and C.

Baby's Dinner Soufflé

⅔ cup Steamed Vegetables (page 46)
⅔ cup cottage cheese
2 heaping tablespoons grated goat cheese (or other soft cheese)
⅓ cup yogurt

Choose any selection of fresh vegetables available such as celery, peas, green beans, squash, onions, carrots, etc. Chop them into bite-sized pieces and steam in vegetable steamer. Set aside. Combine cheeses and yogurt in blender and purée until a smooth paste. Add vegetables and purée until chunky oatmeal consistency is achieved. 2 servings.
Serve from 4 to 6 months on. This makes a good dinner for babies.

Contains protein, calcium, phosphorus, potassium, sodium, vitamins A, B and C.

McFab's Barley Dinner

1 cup vegetable bouillon (Swiss bouillon cubes are good for this)
½ cup hulled barley
½ teaspoon sea salt
¼ cup shredded onion
1 teaspoon finely minced parsley
¼ cup grated carrots
1 tablespoon soybean oleomargarine
2 tablespoons yogurt

Bring bouillon to a boil and add barley and salt very slowly so that the boiling does not stop. Reheat to a full, rolling boil and then lower heat. Let barley simmer 15 minutes and add onion, parsley, carrots and margarine. Let simmer about 8 to 10 minutes longer, and remove from heat. Let cool to lukewarm and put in blender with yogurt. Purée to an oatmeallike consistency. 2 servings.
Serve from 8 months on. This makes a good evening meal.

Contains protein, iron, calcium, phosphorus, potassium, sodium, niacin, vitamins A and C.

Pleasing Peas

¼ cup milk
½ cup fresh peas
¼ cup grated Gouda cheese
 1 heaping tablespoon yogurt

Heat milk in saucepan and add peas. Stir well for a minute or two. Cover and simmer about 8 minutes. Do not allow milk to boil. Remove from heat and add cheese; let stand until lukewarm. Pour into blender and add yogurt. Purée to a smooth, puddinglike texture. 1 serving.
Serve from 6 months on. Good for lunch or dinner.

Contains protein, calcium, phosphorus, potassium, niacin, vitamins A, B and C.

Spinach Soufflé

½ cup cooked spinach
 3 tablespoons yogurt
 3 tablespoons ricotta cheese
 1 teaspoon lemon juice

Combine all ingredients in blender and purée to the consistency of cheese cake. 1 or 2 servings.
Serve from 6 months on. A good, quick dinner.

Contains calcium, phosphorus, potassium, sodium, iron, vitamins A, B and C.

Corn Soufflé

½ cup cooked fresh corn
⅓ cup Cooked Millet (page 44)
 2 tablespoons ricotta cheese
 2 teaspoons honey
    Splash of tomato juice

To cook corn, bring enough water to a boil to entirely cover corn, along with one teaspoon of honey. Remove the husks from corn and drop into boiling water. Return to a boil and turn the heat off. Let corn sit for 5 to 8 minutes. Cut corn from cob and combine with remaining ingredients in blender. Purée to a pudding-like consistency, using more tomato juice if necessary.

Serve from 8 months on. 1 or 2 servings.

Contains protein, potassium, vitamins A and C.

Rutabaga Royale

   1 rutabaga
   ½ cup milk
   1 egg yolk
   1 teaspoon soybean oleomargarine
   1 teaspoon blackstrap molasses
     Freshly grated nutmeg

Peel rutabaga and cut into small pieces. Heat milk in saucepan and add rutabaga. Stir for a few minutes, making sure rutabaga pieces are thoroughly coated with milk. Cover saucepan and let simmer about 20 minutes, or until tender. Stir occasionally while cooking. Remove from heat and let stand until lukewarm. Put in blender with remaining ingredients and purée to the consistency of mashed potatoes. 1 or 2 servings.

Serve from 8 months on.

Contains protein, iron, calcium, phosphorus, potassium, vitamins A, B, C and lecithin.

NOTE: See Chapter V for more dinners for baby.

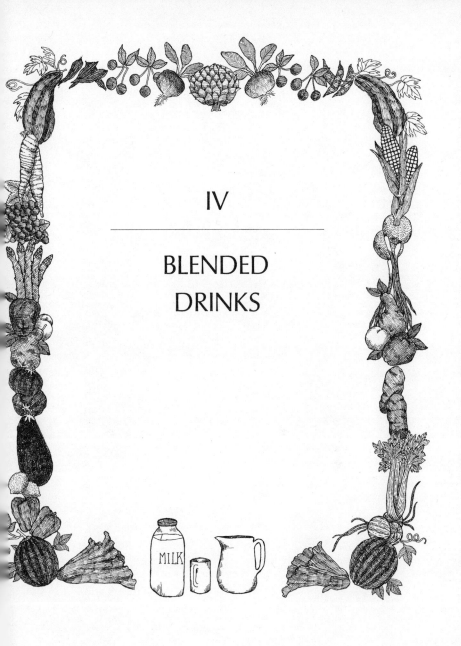

IV

BLENDED
DRINKS

MILK DRINKS

The Basic Formula

    1 baby bottle milk (scalded for younger infants)
    1 level teaspoon to 1 heaping tablespoon brewer's yeast
    ⅓ a banana
    1 teaspoon blackstrap molasses (optional—see below)

Combine all ingredients in blender and liquefy. This recipe, or your own variation of it, is a good formula to start your child on as soon as you begin to wean him from the breast. Start with a level teaspoonful of yeast and gradually build it up to a heaping table-spoonful. The addition of molasses gives this formula more iron, but use with caution, as molasses can give some babies diarrhea. Wait to try the molasses until your baby is at least 9 months old, but dis-continue if loose bowel movements develop. I have found this formula indispensable for a vegetarian child because it is rich in protein, iron and amino acids.

Start this formula from 6 months on. Try, if at all possible, to nurse your child for at least 6 months, the longer the better. There really is no substitute for mother's milk.

Contains protein, iron, calcium, phosphorus, vitamins A, B and C.

Maxie's Malted Milk

    1 cup goat's milk
1½ tablespoons malted milk powder
⅓ cup powdered milk
    1 cup ice cream made with honey
¼ teaspoon vanilla

Combine all ingredients in blender and purée to the consistency of a malted milk. 2 servings.

Serve from 6 months on.

Contains protein, calcium, phosphorus, potassium, vitamins A and B.

Cinnamon Sling

    1 cup milk
    1 cup ice cream made with honey
    1 ripe banana
½ teaspoon cinnamon

Combine all ingredients in blender and purée until rich and creamy. 2 servings.

Serve from 6 months on. This is a good winter party drink for children.

Contains protein, calcium, phosphorus, potassium, vitamins A, B and C.

Baby Eggnog

    1 cup goat's milk
    1 egg yolk
    2 teaspoons honey
¼ cup powdered milk
½ teaspoon vanilla
    Freshly grated nutmeg

Combine all ingredients in blender and purée until well mixed. 1 serving.

Serve from 6 months on. This is a good Christmastime drink for babies and older children.

Contains protein, calcium, lecithin, phosphorus, potassium, vitamins A and B.

St. John's Julep

    1 cup milk
    ½ teaspoon vanilla
    2 heaping tablespoons carob powder
    ½ cup yogurt
    1 teaspoon brewer's yeast (optional)

Combine all ingredients in blender and purée until frothy. 1 serving.

Serve from 4 to 6 months on. This is good to serve a baby in place of an afternoon bottle.

Contains protein, calcium, phosphorus, vitamins A and B.

Strawberry Sunday

    1 cup milk
    1 cup ice cream made with honey
    ½ cup fresh strawberries

Combine all ingredients in blender and purée until creamy. 2 servings.

Serve from 4 to 6 months on. This is a good sweet treat for babies and older children.

Contains protein, calcium, phosphorus, potassium, vitamins A, B and C.

February Frappe

    4 dried figs
    4 dried apricots
    4 cups milk
    ½ cup yogurt
    2 tablespoons blackstrap molasses

Place figs and apricots in blender with 2 cups milk and liquefy until fruit is completely dissolved in the liquid mixture; add remaining ingredients and purée until liquid is frothy. 4 servings.

Serve from 6 months on. Add an egg and you have a quick, complete breakfast for baby.

Contains protein, iron, calcium, phosphorus, potassium, vitamins A, B, niacin and C.

Raisin Shake

    ½ cup raisins
    1 cup apple juice
    2 cups milk
    1 ripe banana
    1 cup yogurt
    2 tablespoons blackstrap molasses

Soften raisins overnight in apple juice; place in blender with any remaining juice and purée until raisins are completely blended; add remaining ingredients and purée again until milkshake consistency is reached. 4 servings.

Serve from 6 months on. This is also a good drink for pregnant women.

Contains protein, calcium, iron, phosphorus, potassium, sodium, vitamins A, B, niacin and C.

Peachy Keen

    1 ripe peach
    1 cup milk
    1 teaspoon honey
    ¼ teaspoon powdered cloves

Chop up peach and combine with remaining ingredients in blender and purée until light and frothy. 1 serving.
Serve from 4 to 6 months on.

Contains protein, calcium, phosphorus, potassium, vitamins A, B and C.

Working Baby Breakfast

  1¼ cups milk
    2 heaping tablespoons cooked oatmeal or farina
    1 ripe banana
    1 tablespoon blackstrap molasses
    1 egg yolk (optional)

Combine all ingredients in blender and liquefy. 2 servings.
Serve from 4 to 6 months on for a breakfast quickie.

Contains protein, calcium, iron, phosphorus, potassium, sodium, vitamins A, B and C.

Early September

    5 dried apricots in apricot nectar to cover
    1 medium yellow summer squash
    2 cups milk
    1 teaspoon honey

Soak apricots in nectar overnight in refrigerator to soften; pour into blender. Chop squash and add with remaining ingredients to blender. Liquefy until milkshake consistency is achieved. 2 to 3 servings.

Serve from 4 to 6 months on. A good all-around liquid meal.

Contains protein, calcium, iron, phosphorus, potassium, sodium, vitamins A, B and C.

Palermo's Drink

    1 apple
    ½ cup milk
    ½ cup yogurt
    4 tablespoons carob powder

Core apple and leave unpeeled; chop and combine in blender with remaining ingredients. Purée to the consistency of a milkshake. 1 or 2 servings.

Serve from 4 to 6 months on. This is good for a liquid lunch.

Contains protein, calcium, phosphorus, potassium, vitamins A, B, C and lecithin.

Winter's Morn

    3 dried apricots in apple juice to cover
    1 apple
 1½ cups milk
    1 ripe banana
    1 tablespoon brewer's yeast

Soak apricots in apple juice overnight in refrigerator. Put in blender with any remaining liquid. Core apple and chop in small pieces; add to blender with remaining ingredients and liquefy. 2 to 3 servings.

Serve from 4 to 6 months on as a quick breakfast drink.

Contains protein, iron, phosphorus, potassium, sodium, vitamins A, B, niacin and C.

Bright Tiger Drink

    1½ cups milk
     1 tablespoon Tiger's Milk
    ½ a ripe banana
    ¼ cup shredded coconut
     1 teaspoon brewer's yeast (optional)

Combine all ingredients in blender and liquefy to the consistency of a milkshake. 1 to 2 servings.
Serve from 6 months on.

Contains protein, calcium, phosphorus, potassium, vitamins A, B and C.

Max's First Date

    1 cup milk
    4 pitted dates
  ½ cup yogurt
    1 teaspoon honey
  ⅓ teaspoon cinnamon

Combine all ingredients in blender and purée until frothy. 2 servings.
Serve from 6 months on. Good for a quick winter breakfast or lunch.

Contains iron, calcium, phosphorus, potassium, vitamins A and B.

Screwdriver Special

  1 medium ripe tomato
  1 cup milk
  1 cup tomato juice
  1 teaspoon Tamari soy sauce
  1 tablespoon brewer's yeast

Chop tomato and combine with remaining ingredients in blender. Liquefy until completely dissolved. 2 servings.

Serve from 6 months on. Easy way to serve a vegetable.

Contains protein, iron, calcium, phosphorus, potassium, sodium, vitamins A, B and C.

FRUIT AND YOGURT DRINKS

Summer Quickie

- ¾ cup fresh bing cherries
- 3 ripe plums
- ½ cup fresh blueberries
  Juice of ½ lime
- 1½ cups apricot nectar

Pit cherries; chop plums coarsely. Combine cherries and plums with blueberries in the blender. Add lime juice and nectar and liquefy until milklike texture is reached. 3 servings.

Serve from 6 months on as a liquid lunch or to older children as a snack.

VARIATION: Take ½ cup of this mixture and a heaping ¼ cup cottage cheese and purée in blender. Pour over cereal and add milk for a complete breakfast or lunch.

Contains calcium, phosphorus, potassium, vitamins A and C.

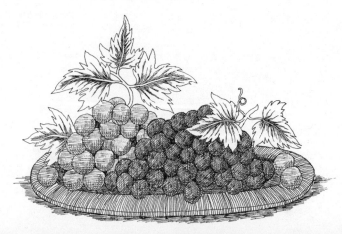

Breakfast-Plus Booster Drink
(a *great* family drink)

    1 quart fresh orange juice
    4 tablespoons brewer's yeast
    1 large ripe banana
    2 tablespoons blackstrap molasses

Liquefy all ingredients in blender until milkshake consistency
is reached. 4 servings.

Serve from 4 to 6 months on. Serve this also to busy adults as a
high-protein breakfast drink. Also good on reducing diet as substitute for a meal.

VARIATION: Combine 1 cup of Booster Drink with ½ cup yogurt
and serve to baby as liquid breakfast. Very good for hot days or
hassled mornings.

Contains protein, calcium, iron, potassium, sodium, vitamins A,
B, niacin and C.

Phoenician New Year's Drink

    1 baby bottle freshly squeezed orange juice
       Juice of ½ lemon
    2 teaspoons parsley leaves
       Vitamin C tablet, crushed*

Combine all ingredients in blender and purée. I gave this drink
to my son often during the long winter months. Parsley is an extra-
nutritious green vegetable with amazingly high amounts of protein,
iron and vitamin A. The orange juice, lemon juice and vitamin C
provide a potent remedy for the winter cold blues. Makes 1 serving.

Serve from 9 months on.

Contains protein, calcium, phosphorus, iron, vitamins A and C.

---

* Use under 100 mg. for children under 1 year old; use 250 to 500 mg. for
children over 1 year old. Consult your own pediatrician for dosage best suited
for your own child.

December Morning Quickie

> 1 cup fresh orange juice
> ½ cup water
> ⅓ ripe banana
> 1 heaping teaspoon cashew butter
> 1 heaping teaspoon Abby Van Derek's Incredible Granola (page 32)
> 1 teaspoon brewer's yeast
> 1 tablespoon Tiger's Milk

Combine all ingredients in blender and purée until a milkshake consistency is reached. 1 or 2 servings.

Serve from 4 to 6 months on. A good liquid breakfast.

Contains protein, iron, calcium, phosphorus, potassium, sodium, vitamins A, B, niacin and C.

Summertime Exotica

> ½ ripe papaya
> 10 to 15 pitted bing cherries
> 10 strawberries
> 1 cup yogurt

Scoop out papaya, discarding seeds, and combine with cherries and strawberries in blender. Add yogurt and purée in blender until foamy. 2 servings.

Serve from 4 to 6 months on as a quick lunch or afternoon refresher.

VARIATION: Add 2 cups apple juice to drink, stir well, and serve to entire family as punch.

Contains protein, calcium, phosphorus, potassium, sodium, vitamins A, B and C.

Cool Cantaloupe Drink

      ½ cantaloupe
      ½ cup yogurt
      ⅔ cup lemonade (sugarless)
      2 teaspoons honey

Scoop out cantaloupe and combine in blender with remaining ingredients. Liquefy to milkshake consistency. 2 servings.

Serve from 4 to 6 months on as liquid lunch. Good for hot days when babies reject solids.

Contains protein, calcium, phosphorus, potassium, sodium, vitamins A, B and C.

Summer Punch à la Max

      1 cup scooped-out Cranshaw melon
      1 cup scooped-out watermelon
      2 cups apple juice

Combine all ingredients in blender and liquefy until foamy. 3 or 4 servings.

Serve from 4 to 6 months on. Good for hot afternoons.

Contains calcium, phosphorus, potassium, sodium, vitamins A and C.

Red Currant Cocktail

      4 dried pear halves
      ⅛ cup raisins
      3 cups red currant juice (if not available, use cranberry juice)
      1 cup yogurt
      4 heaping teaspoons brewer's yeast

Soak pears and raisins overnight in currant juice to cover. Place in blender and liquefy. Add remaining ingredients and purée until frothy. 4 servings.

Serve from 6 months on. Makes a complete meal anytime.

Contains protein, iron, calcium, phosphorus, potassium, vitamin A, B and C.

Rosy Raspberry Morning

1 ripe peach
2 cups fresh raspberries
1 cup yogurt
1 cup peach nectar

Chop up peach and combine with remaining ingredients in blender; purée until milkshake consistency is reached. 4 servings.

Serve from 6 months on. This makes a good topping for breakfast cereal or a cool summer-afternoon drink.

Contains protein, calcium, phosphorus, potassium, vitamins A, B and C.

Cold Prevention Drink

⅔ cup fresh orange juice
⅓ cup water
2 dried apricot halves
1 100 mg. rose-hips vitamin C tablet*

Combine all ingredients in blender and purée until frothy. 1 serving.

Serve from 6 months on. Good to serve if you suspect your child might be coming down with a cold.

Contains calcium, potassium, sodium, vitamins A and C.

* After 1 year of age, use 500 mg. vitamin C.

Cranacot Drink

⅔ cup Cooked Cranberries (page 65)
5 teaspoons apricot concentrate
1 teaspoon brewer's yeast
½ cup water

Combine all ingredients and liquefy in blender. 1 serving.
Serve from 6 months on.

Contains protein, calcium, phosphorus, potassium, vitamins A, B, C and niacin.

Another Drink

½ apple
½ cup Cooked Cranberries (page 65)
½ ripe banana
½ cup apple juice

Core and chop apple, but leave unpeeled. Combine with remaining ingredients in blender and purée to a rich thick consistency. 1 or 2 servings.
Serve from 6 months on.

Contains calcium, potassium, vitamins A and C.

Blueberry Summer Cooler

½ cantaloupe
1 ripe peach
¾ cup fresh blueberries
1 teaspoon honey
1½ cups yogurt

Scoop out cantaloupe, discarding seeds, cut up and put in blender; include all juices. Cut up peach and add, with remaining ingredients, to blender. Liquefy until milklike texture is achieved. 2 or 3 servings.

Serve from 4 to 6 months on and continue serving throughout childhood.

Contains protein, calcium, phosphorus, potassium, vitamins A, B and C.

The Grand Grape Drink

    15 to 20 fresh green grapes
     1 medium-size ripe banana
     1 teaspoon honey (optional)
     1 cup yogurt
    ½ cup milk

Combine all ingredients in blender and liquefy until foamy. 2 servings.

Serve from 4 to 6 months on. Good for lunch.

Contains protein, calcium, phosphorus, potassium, vitamins A, B and C.

Early One Morning

    ¾ cup yogurt
    ¾ cup apple juice
     4 kiwi fruits
     1 whole honeydew melon

Cut kiwi fruit in half and scoop out pulp; put pulp in blender. Scoop out honeydew melon, discarding seeds, and add to kiwi-fruit pulp in blender. Include all juices. Add remaining ingredients and liquefy until frothy. 2 or 3 servings.

Serve from 4 to 6 months on as hot-weather lunch and to the whole family as a summer punch.

Contains protein, calcium, phosphorus, potassium, vitamins A, B and C.

Apricot Malt

   8 to 10 dried apricots
   3 cups apple juice
   1 ripe banana
   1 cup yogurt
   2 tablespoons brewer's yeast (optional)

Put apricots in blender with 1 cup apple juice and purée until apricots are completely dissolved into a creamy nectar. Add remaining ingredients and liquefy until foamy. 4 servings.

Serve from 4 to 6 months on. This is a good winter meal, as dried fruits and bananas are always available. Also use this drink with yeast as a good liquid meal for adult dieters. Drink one 8-ounce glass in place of one meal a day (preferably dinner).

Contains protein, calcium, phosphorus, potassium, vitamins A, B and C.

Apricot November

   8 dried apricots
   2 fresh peaches or 4 dried peaches
   1 quart fresh orange juice
   1 cup yogurt
*1 tablespoon safflower oil (optional)

Put apricots in blender with 1 cup orange juice and purée until creamy; add peaches and 1 cup orange juice and purée again until all fruit is completely dissolved. Add remaining orange juice and yogurt and stir until completely mixed. 4 servings.

Serve from 4 to 6 months on. An easy winter drink.

   * For women: Add the safflower oil and make a drink that's good for women who need a fresher-looking skin. Every morning drink an 8-ounce glass in place of other food. Wear no cosmetics whatsoever, except a light moisturizer, if desired. Wash face twice daily with tawashi (Japanese dried-seaweed sponge, good for revitalizing the skin) or rough-textured terry-cloth washcloth and pure castile soap. Continue this routine for 2 weeks.

Contains protein, calcium, phosphorus, potassium, vitamins A, B and C.

Accord Summer Drink

1 whole honeydew melon
1 cup yogurt
1 cup apricot nectar
¾ cup pitted bing cherries
¾ cup blueberries

Scoop out honeydew melon, discarding seeds. Put in blender with all juices. Add remaining ingredients and liquefy in blender until frothy. 4 servings.

Serve from 4 to 6 months on as lunch or summer punch.

Contains protein, calcium, phosphorus, potassium, vitamins A, B and C.

Bright and Early

1 papaya
1 whole cantaloupe
2 teaspoons honey
1 cup yogurt
½ cup pear nectar
½ cup cranberry juice

Scoop out papaya and cantaloupe, discarding seeds. Put in blender, including all juices. Add remaining ingredients and liquefy until foamy. 3 to 4 servings.

Serve from 4 to 6 months on as liquid breakfast or lunch. Serve to entire family as a breakfast booster drink.

Contains protein, calcium, lecithin, phosphorus, potassium, sodium, vitamins A, B and C.

10 A.M. Powerhouse

  ½ fresh tangerine, peeled
  1 heaping tablespoon Tiger's Milk
  1 apple, cored and peeled
  4 tablespoons yogurt
  4 tablespoons Abby Van Derek's Incredible Granola (page 32)
     Splash of milk

Divide tangerine into segments; combine with remaining ingredients in blender, using enough milk to keep mixture to the consistency of a heavy milkshake. Purée until thoroughly mixed. 1 or 2 servings.

Serve from 4 to 6 months on. A good morning booster drink.

Contains protein, calcium, phosphorus, potassium, sodium, vitamins A, B, niacin and C.

Springtime Sling

  ½ cup fresh grated carrot
  2 cups fresh orange juice
  3 teaspoons raisins
1½ teaspoons honey

Conbine all ingredients in blender and liquefy to a creamy, milkshake texture. 2 servings.

Serve from 6 months on. A lovely lunch.

Contains phosphorus, potassium, sodium, vitamins A and C.

Mr. Baby's Blackberry Julep

  1 cup fresh blackberries
  ½ cup fresh pineapple, chopped
  1 cup yogurt
  1 cup grape juice

Combine all ingredients in blender and purée to a milkshake consistency. 3 servings.

Serve from 6 months on. Good as an afternoon cooler for baby or poured over a fruit compote to serve the entire family.

Contains protein, calcium, phosphorus, potassium, vitamins A, B and C.

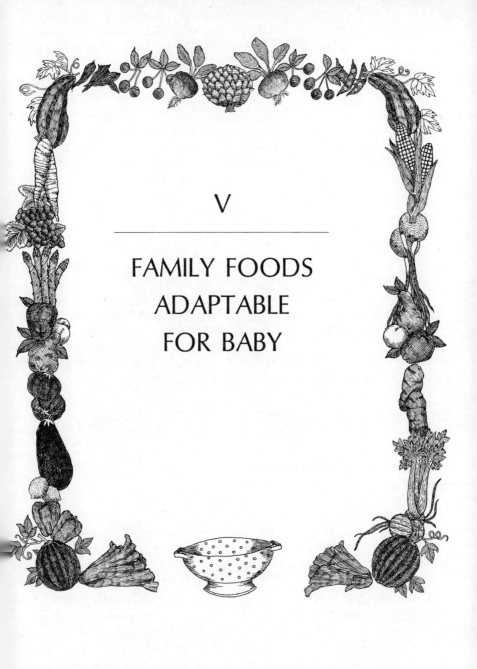

V

FAMILY FOODS
ADAPTABLE
FOR BABY

MAIN COURSE DISHES

To bed, to bed, says Sleepy-Head;
Let's stay awhile, says Slow
Put on the pan, says Greedy Ann
We'll sup before we go.
—MOTHER GOOSE

New Mexican Pueblo Bread

  2 cups pine nuts (piñón nuts)*
  ¾ cup lukewarm water
  ½ teaspoon sea salt
     Corn oil

In a blender, grind nuts to a coarse meal. Transfer to a mixing bowl and mix well with the water and salt. Let stand at room temperature for at least 2 hours. Liberally grease a large skillet or griddle with oil. Drop the nut mixture onto the griddle by the tablespoonful and pat with your hands into a well-shaped 3½-inch-wide patty. Brown slowly on each side, about 10 to 15 minutes for each side. Turn patties with a very well oiled turner, as the mixture tends to stick. Patties should be brown and slightly crusty on the outside. Makes 6 patties.

---

* Piñón nuts, or pine nuts, as they are called in many parts of this country, have been an important food to the Indians of the Southwest since before 1536, when they were first introduced by the Indians to Spanish explorers. Today it is generally accepted that this native American nut surpasses the European pignolia in both nutritive value and delicate taste. The piñón nut is obtained from the cone of some species of pine trees, the most useful of which is the *Pinus edulis*. New Mexico is the best source of piñón nuts. For ordering piñón nuts and other locally grown Indian foods, write Box 852, San Juan Pueblo, New Mexico.

Serve from 8 months on. This is a fantastic food in your diet as well. It's incredibly easy and quick to prepare, has a high protein count, and a lovely fragrant flavor. It's good for a teething baby to gnaw on, and babies with a few teeth love to chew on it. It's good served for breakfast with poached eggs or for dinner with a soufflé and salad.

Contains protein, iron, vitamins B and C.

Piñón Loaf

> 1 cup pine nuts (piñón nuts)
> 1 tablespoon vegetable oil
> ¼ cup walnuts
> 1 egg, beaten
> 1 Spanish onion, finely chopped
> 1 pound spinach, cooked and cold
> 1 clove garlic
> 1 cup whole wheat bread crumbs
> ½ teaspoon sea salt
> ⅓ teaspoon sage

First, over medium heat, sauté piñón nuts in about 1 tablespoon oil until well browned on all sides, stirring continually. This takes about 15 minutes.

Preheat oven to 350° F.

In a blender, gradually combine all nuts, egg, onion, spinach and garlic. Blend until smooth. In a mixing bowl, combine bread crumbs, salt, and sage. Add nut-spinach purée and mix thoroughly. Turn into a well-oiled loaf pan and bake for 30 minutes. 6 servings.

Serve from 8 months on. A good dinner dish.

Contains protein, calcium, phosphorus, lecithin, iron, vitamins A and C.

Burgie Delight or Soyball Sensation

6 tablespoons sesame oil
1 large Spanish onion, chopped
2 cups Cooked Soybeans (page 41)
½ cup grated Gouda cheese
2 eggs, well beaten
1 cup peanuts
½ cup whole wheat or rye bread crumbs
1 tablespoon Tamari soy sauce
1 large clove garlic

Heat about 2 tablespoons oil and add onion. Sauté until wilted and browned, about 15 to 20 minutes. Add a bit of water to onions for moisture, if necessary, as they cook. Combine cooked onions with soybeans, cheese, eggs and peanuts. Grind well in a blender or put through a food chopper using fine blade. (When your baby begins to chew well, or if you are making this for adults, blend to a chunkier texture.) Pour into mixing bowl and work in bread crumbs and Tamari soy sauce. Shape into patties. Mince clove of garlic and heat 4 tablespoons oil in large skillet. Add garlic and stir until garlic is lightly browned. Add patties and sauté over a medium heat until nicely browned on both sides, about 15 minutes on each side. 4 to 6 patties.

Serve from 6 months on. This is an excellent dinner for vegetarian babies. Mash up pattie for a baby with no teeth; moisten a bit with milk or tomato juice, if necessary. When a child is ready to begin feeding himself, cut the patties into small squares and let him help himself. Serve to school-age children on a toasted roll with lettuce, tomato and mayonnaise.

VARIATION: Shape batter into walnut-sized balls and sauté as above. Serve with Parsley Spaghetti (page 129) or buttered spinach noodles. With a chilled bottle of white wine and your own fresh fruit compote, this makes a lovely light dinner.

Contains protein, calcium, phosphorus, iron, vitamins A, B, C and lecithin.

Soy Sandwich Spread

    1 cup Cooked Soybeans (page 41)
    1 tablespoon finely minced onion
    2 tablespoons finely chopped pimento *or*
    1 tablespoon finely chopped dill pickle
    2 tablespoons finely chopped celery
    ½ teaspoon caraway seeds
    1 to 2 tablespoons mayonnaise

Mash up the soybeans with a fork until they're approximately ¾ mashed and ¼ whole bean. Combine with the remaining ingredients and keep chilled in the refrigerator. Makes about 1½ cups spread.

Serve from 1 year on—purée in the blender, if necessary. This spread makes delicious sandwiches, particularily if made on rye bread with a layer of crisp lettuce. This recipe will come in very handy if you have to send your children off with a packed lunch.

Contains protein, calcium, iron, phosphorus, potassium, vitamins A, B, C and lecithin.

Anna's Manna—Broiled Soyburgers

    4 to 6 tablespoons safflower oil
    1 large Spanish onion, finely minced
    2 tablespoons Tamari soy sauce
    ⅔ cup carrots, finely grated
    4 tablespoons pine nuts, ground
    2 cups Cooked Soybeans (page 41)
    2 eggs, beaten
    4 to 6 tablespoons dry whole wheat bread crumbs

Heat about 4 tablespoons oil in skillet and add onion. Sauté until wilted and browned, about 15 to 20 minutes. Stir frequently. Add soy sauce during the last 3 minutes of cooking. Remove onions from pan and set aside. Add remaining 2 tablespoons of oil to skillet and heat. Add carrots and pine nuts and sauté, stirring frequently, for about 10 to 15 minutes. Set aside. In a blender, combine soybeans, eggs and onions. Purée until soybeans are completely dissolved. Pour into a mixing bowl and add carrot-pine nut mixture and bread crumbs. Stir well. Shape into patties and place on an oiled cookie sheet. Place under broiler and cook for about 15 minutes on each side, or until patties are nicely browned. 6 patties.

Serve from 6 months on. This makes a wonderful main course for vegetarian babies because of its high protein content. You can spoon-feed this to young babies. Mash a bit, if necessary, or moisten with a dash of tomato juice. When the child is ready for "finger foods," use whole pine nuts instead of ground ones. Cut the patties into small squares and let baby help himself.

VARIATION: Serve soyburgers to the whole family. After they're broiled, grate some Cheddar cheese over the top and place under broiler for a few seconds to melt the cheese. Serve on a hamburger roll with lettuce, tomato and mayonnaise.

Contains protein, calcium, lecithin, phosphorus, iron, vitamins A, B and C.

Apple Annie's Tomato Sauce and Soybean Casserole

SAUCE

> 2 tablespoons safflower oil
> 1 large Spanish onion, chopped
> 2 apples, unpeeled and chopped
>   Dash of apple juice
> 1 cup tomato paste
> 1 cup water
> 4 tomatoes, finely chopped
> 3 tablespoons raw wheat germ
>   Sea salt to taste

In a skillet heat the oil and add the onion. Sauté, stirring frequently, until onion begins to brown, about 15 minutes.

In a blender, purée the apples with enough juice to facilitate blending, until they dissolve into a saucelike consistency.

Combine onions, apples and remaining ingredients in a heavy saucepan; bring to a boil, cover, and reduce heat to a slow simmer. Simmer for 2½ to 3 hours. Let the sauce stand for at least 1 hour (the longer the better) before serving.

CASSEROLE

> 2 tablespoons safflower oil
> 3 cups broccoli flowerets
> 2½ tablespoons Tamari soy sauce
> 2½ cups Cooked Soybeans (page 41)
> 2 cups grated Cheddar cheese, firmly packed

In a wok or skillet, heat the oil and add the broccoli; sauté over high heat, stirring continually, for 1 minute. Add the soy sauce and cook for another minute or two. Make sure that the soy sauce is distributed evenly over the broccoli. Set aside.

In a 2-quart casserole dish, make 1 layer of soybeans, then cheese and sauce. Then add a layer of broccoli, cheese and sauce. Alternate until ingredients are used up. Top casserole with a sprinkling of cheese and bake at 350° F., covered, for 20 to 25 minutes. 6 servings.

Serve from 8 months on—just purée the finished dish in the blender for babies who can't chew well yet. This one casserole provides enough nutrients in itself to be a complete meal. It's hearty and delicious and well worth making a regular item in your menu.

Contains protein, iron, calcium, sodium, phosphorus, potassium, lecithin, vitamins A, B, C and E.

Eastern Casserole

> 1 cup brown rice
> 1 cup lentils
> 5 tablespoons blackstrap molasses
> 4 tablespoons Tamari soy sauce
> ½ cup coarsely chopped hazelnuts (or walnuts)
> 2 Spanish onions

2 green peppers
Safflower oil for sautéing
Juice of ½ lemon
Juice of ½ lime
4 tablespoons grated sharp Cheddar cheese

Steam rice and lentils together (page 42). Set aside and add molasses, soy sauce and hazelnuts. Chop onions and peppers and sauté in safflower oil until completely wilted and slightly browned, about ½ hour. While sautéing, sprinkle occasionally with a bit of soy sauce and juice of lemon and lime. Add this to rice-lentil combination and mix. Top with grated cheese and set under broiler for a few moments until cheese is melted and browned. Serve warm. 4 servings.

Serve from 6 months on, just mashing slightly or grinding in blender for small baby. This is a good winter dinner for the entire family. And it's even better the second day.

VARIATION: For a hearty breakfast, warm leftover casserole and place a small to medium-sized portion on plate, topped with two poached eggs.

Contains protein, iron, calcium, phosphorus, potassium, sodium, lecithin, vitamins A, B, C and E.

Indian Summer Dinner

2 large Spanish onions
6 tablespoons corn oil
4 tablespoons Tamari soy sauce
2 cups Cooked Rice and Lentils (page 42)
⅔ cup mung bean sprouts
5 tablespoons crumbled feta cheese

Chop onions coarsely. Heat oil in skillet and add onions. Sauté until onions are wilted and browned, about 20 minutes. Stir frequently. Add Tamari soy sauce and stir well. Add rice and lentils and mix well with onions. Sauté a few more minutes. Add sprouts and cheese and sauté only until cheese begins to melt, 2 or 3 minutes. 3 or 4 servings.

Serve from 8 months on. Purée in blender with a dash of tomato juice. This makes a good summer dinner served with a tossed green salad and fresh fruits.

Contains protein, iron, calcium, phosphorus, vitamins A, B, C and lecithin.

Lentil Loaf à la Damascus

½ pound Cheddar cheese
2 cups cooked lentils
½ Spanish onion
½ teaspoon salt
¼ teaspoon thyme
1 cup soft whole wheat bread crumbs, packed firmly
1 egg, slightly beaten
1 tablespoon safflower oil

Grind together cheese, lentils and onion. Add salt and thyme. Mix in bread crumbs, egg and oil. Work together thoroughly. Bake in a greased loaf pan at 350° F. for 45 minutes. Serve with Eggplant Florence Sauce (page 119). 4 servings.

Serve from 8 months on. Just mash slightly or combine with yogurt in blender and purée. This makes a good dinner entrée for a winter night; serve with Onion-Prune Pzazz (page 137) and salad of crisp greens.

Contains protein, sodium, phosphorus, vitamins A, B, C and lecithin.

Lentil Salad

2 cups cooked lentils
2 tablespoons lemon juice
3 tablespoons corn oil

1 Spanish onion, minced
½ cup parsley, minced
4 tomatoes, quartered

Combine lentils, lemon juice, oil and onion; let stand for 3 or 4 hours. At serving time, toss with parsley and garnish with tomatoes. 4 servings.

Serve from 1 year on. Purée in blender with a bit of yogurt. This makes a good summer luncheon salad.

Contains protein, iron, lecithin, sodium, phosphorus, vitamins A, B and C.

Barley-Nut Casserole

½ cup pine nuts (piñón variety is the best—see page 110)
2 tablespoons soybean oleomargarine
½ cup safflower oil
1 medium Spanish onion, coarsely chopped
½ pound mushrooms, sliced
4 stalks celery, sliced thinly on the diagonal
1 cup barley
4 cups vegetable bouillon
1½ tablespoons Tamari soy sauce

Preheat oven to 350° F.

Heat margarine in a skillet and add pine nuts. Sauté, stirring frequently, until nuts are browned on all sides. Remove from skillet and set aside.

Heat oil in a large skillet and add onion. Sauté for about 10 minutes, stirring frequently. Add mushrooms, celery and barley and sauté for another 10 minutes, stirring frequently. Add nuts, bouillon and soy sauce and bring to a boil.

Pour into a casserole and bake, covered, for 1 hour and 15 minutes, or until barley is tender and the bouillon is absorbed. 6 servings.

Serve from 8 months on. Just purée in blender.

Contains protein, calcium, phosphorus, iron, lecithin, vitamins A, B, C and E.

Arizona Eggplant

> 1 large eggplant
> 4 medium zucchini squash
> 2 eggs, well beaten
> Safflower oil for sautéing
> 1 large Spanish onion
> 2 tablespoons Tamari soy sauce
> 1½ cups tomato paste
> 1 cup water
> 1 teaspoon honey
> 1 teaspoon oregano
> 1 teaspoon salt
> 4 cups sliced fresh mushrooms
> 1 pound ricotta cheese
> ⅓ to ½ cup Burgundy wine

Peel eggplant and slice into rounds, about ⅓ inch wide. Leave zucchini squash unpeeled and cut into halves lengthwise; then slice into pieces about ⅓ inch wide. Heat about two tablespoons corn oil in a large skillet; dip eggplant slices into beaten egg and brown in oil, about 3 minutes on each side. Add more oil as you go along, if necessary. Set eggplant aside on paper toweling to drain off excess oil. Repeat process with zucchini.

Chop onion in small pieces and sauté in oil until wilted and browned, about 15 to 20 minutes. Stir frequently. Add soy sauce during the last 5 minutes of cooking. In a heavy saucepan combine onions, tomato paste, water, honey, oregano and salt. Bring to a boil and reduce heat. Cover and simmer slowly for about 40 minutes. Meanwhile, sauté the mushrooms in oil for about 3 to 5 minutes, or until barely cooked. Add mushrooms and ricotta cheese to the sauce and remove from heat. Add the wine to the sauce, using more or less depending on how thick you like your sauce.

In an oiled casserole dish, arrange one layer of eggplant, top with sauce, then a layer of zucchini, and more sauce. Continue process until all ingredients are used. Bake at 350° F. for 30 minutes. 4 servings.

Serve from 8 months on. To serve a baby whose teeth haven't

come in yet, just purée in the blender, or mash with a fork. This is a good food to serve as is to a baby who does have a few teeth. Simply cut into small pieces.

Contains protein, calcium, lecithin, potassium, vitamins A, B, C and E.

Eggplant Florence

SAUCE

> Safflower oil for sautéing
> 1 clove garlic, finely minced
> 1 large Spanish onion, chopped medium fine
> ½ cup water
> 3 cups fresh tomatoes, finely chopped
> 1 green pepper, finely chopped
> 1 cup tomato paste
> 2 teaspoons dried mint leaves
> Salt and pepper to taste

Heat safflower oil in skillet; add garlic and sauté for a few seconds, until lightly browned; add onion and sauté over a low flame until gently browned and wilted (about 45 to 60 minutes)—add ½ cup water, a little at a time, while cooking, and stir onions occasionally. Add tomatoes, pepper, tomato paste, mint, salt and pepper; cover and cook over a low flame until a rich sauce is formed, about 30 minutes. Let sauce sit for at least 2 hours before using.

EGGPLANT

> 1 large eggplant
> 3 medium or 2 large zucchini squash
> Safflower oil for sautéing
> 3 eggs, beaten
> 1½ cups grated Cheddar cheese, tightly packed
> Eggplant Florence Sauce (above)

Peel eggplant and slice into rounds, about ⅓ inch wide. Leave zucchini squash unpeeled and cut into halves lengthwise; then slice into strips about ⅓ inch wide. Heat oil in skillet; dip eggplant slices into beaten egg and brown in oil, adding more oil as you go if necessary. Set eggplant aside, draining off excess oil on paper toweling. Repeat process with zucchini. In an oiled casserole dish, arrange 1 layer of eggplant; top with sauce and sprinkle with cheese. Add a layer of zucchini, sauce and cheese; repeat process until all slices are used. Bake at 350° F. for about 30 minutes. 4 to 6 servings.

Serve from 8 months on. To serve a baby, just mash with a fork. This is a good main dish, served with Simple Simon's Salad (page 150) and a good bottle of red wine.

VARIATION: Pour Eggplant Florence Sauce over a cheese omelet for a good brunch dish.

Contains protein, calcium, potassium, sodium, lecithin, vitamins A, B, C and E.

Gig's Spinach Pie

THE CRUST:

   1 cup unbleached white flour
     or
   1 cup whole wheat *pastry* flour
  ¾ teaspoon sea salt
  ¼ cup safflower oil
  2 tablespoons milk

Place the flour in a mixing bowl with the salt and pour oil and milk over the flour all at once. Mix together with a fork until throughly blended. Roll out between 2 sheets of wax paper on a surface that has been sprinkled with water. This prevents the paper from sliding around too much while you're rolling it out. Now place the crust in a 9-inch pie pan and set aside while you make the filling.

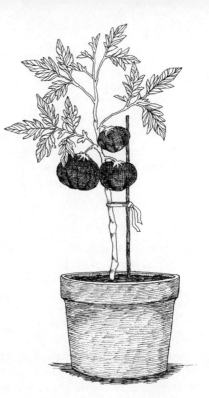

THE FILLING:

1½ pounds fresh spinach
¼ cup chopped onions
2 tablespoons safflower oil
2 eggs
1 cup yogurt
½ cup dry milk
½ teaspoon nutmeg
½ teaspoon sea salt
⅓ cup grated cheese—Gruyère, Parmesan, Swiss, etc.

Wash the spinach well and remove all the stems. Drop spinach in boiling water and cook for a few minutes, or until it goes limp. Drain the spinach well and chop it up. Heat oil in a skillet and add the onions and spinach. Cook for a few minutes, until liquid has evaporated. In a mixing bowl beat the eggs; add yogurt, milk and seasonings. Mix well and add spinach and onions. Stir together and pour into the pie shell; sprinkle with cheese and bake at 375° F. for 25 minutes. Makes 4 servings.

Serve from 6 months on. Just remove the filling from a piece of the pie and mash up very fine; or purée in the blender for a small infant. Babies usually like to gnaw on the crust, too. This makes a wonderful year-round dinner; it's light enough for warm summer evenings and good served cold, too. Serve with a chilled fresh fruit compote and a light, dry white wine.

Contains protein, calcium, iron, phosphorus, vitamins A, B and C.

Chili Non Carne

> 4 tablespoons corn oil
> 2 medium-sized cloves garlic, minced
> 2 medium-sized onions, chopped
> 2 green peppers, chopped
> 2½ cups Cooked Kidney Beans (page 45)
> 2 cups tomato soup
> 1 cup tomato purée
> ½ cup wheat flakes
> ½ cup sesame meal
> ½ cup bulgur wheat
> 1 teaspoon chili powder
> 1½ teaspoons chili con carne seasoning
> 1 teaspoon oregano
> 2 cups water

In a skillet, heat the oil and add garlic; sauté until the garlic begins to brown, and add the onions and peppers. Sauté, stirring frequently, until the onions turn transparent, about 10 to 12 minutes.

In a soup kettle combine onion-pepper mixture with the remaining ingredients. Bring to the edge of a boil, cover and reduce the heat. Simmer slowly for about 1 hour. Turn off the heat and let stand for at least one hour before serving. 6 to 8 servings.

Serve this from 9 months on; just mash slightly and combine with yogurt and a little tomato juice to take the edge off the chili seasonings for a child's more sensitive palate.

Contains protein, calcium, iron, phosphorus, potassium, vitamins A, B, C and E.

Refried Beans (Frijoles Refritos)

> 2½ tablespoons corn oil
> 1 clove garlic, minced
> 1 large Spanish onion, minced
> 2 cups Cooked Pinto Beans, mashed (page 44)

1 hot chili pepper, finely chopped*
2 tablespoons whole wheat flour
6 tablespoons grated Cheddar cheese

In a large skillet, heat the oil. Add the garlic and sauté until garlic begins to brown. Add the onion and cook, stirring frequently, until the onion begins to brown, about 15 to 20 minutes. Add beans, pepper and flour and cook together for 10 to 15 minutes. Add the cheese and cook long enough to melt the cheese. 3 to 4 servings.
Serve from 8 months on.

Contains protein, calcium, phosphorus, vitamins A, B and C.

* Omit the chili pepper if serving to babies or small children.

Tostadas

4   Tortillas (page 41)
2½   cups Refried Beans (page 122)
4   tablespoons grated Cheddar cheese
4   tablespoons shredded lettuce
4   tablespoons finely chopped tomatoes

On each tortilla, spread ½ cup of refried beans; then add cheese, lettuce and tomato. Serve warm. Makes 4 tostadas.
Serve as soon as baby is manipulative enough to hold onto a spoon. Just break off a bit of the tortilla, and let him feed himself.

Contains protein, calcium, phosphorus, vitamins A, B and C.

Canyon de Chelly Casserole

8   chili peppers, roasted
     Safflower oil for sautéing and roasting
4   large ripe tomatoes
     Dried basil for sprinkling
⅔   pound sharp Cheddar cheese (approximately)
4   cups Refried Beans (page 122)

To roast chili peppers, use fairly large peppers (about 2 inches across and 4 inches long). Oil their skins well. Place peppers in a shallow oiled baking pan and roast at 350° F. for 30 to 40 minutes, or until the peppers are soft. If you want the peppers to be less hot, remove all seeds before roasting. During the winter fresh hot peppers are often unobtainable; you may substitute canned green chili peppers, usually available in the Mexican food section of your local grocery. The best peppers come from the Southwestern section of the United States where they are harvested and dried in large quantities during the fall and strung in long, fiery-red bunches outside the adobe dwellings of many New Mexican pueblos. (For Indian-grown chili peppers and other Southwestern speciality groceries, write Box 852, San Juan Pueblo, New Mexico, 87566.)

Slice the tomatoes into ⅓-inch slices; heat oil in a skillet and add the tomatoes. Sprinkle lightly with the basil; turn after about 3 to 4 minutes, sprinkle lightly with basil again, and sauté the other side.

Meanwhile, stuff the roasted chili peppers with cheese cut into ⅓-inch-wide strips and arrange them in a layer to cover the bottom of an oiled 2-quart casserole dish. Then add a layer of the sautéed tomatoes and a layer of the refried beans; continue to layer in this manner until all the ingredients are used up. (This usually means two layers of each separate ingredient.) Top the casserole with some grated Cheddar cheese, cover and bake at 350° F. for 20 to 25 minutes. Makes 6 servings.

Serve this from 1 year on. Just mash slightly. This dish is not so hot as may appear to the reader unaware of Southwestern cuisine. With unseeded peppers, it's quite mild, and my son ate it easily from one year on. This hearty casserole makes for very fine cold-weather dining. Serve it hot with a salad of very crisp, chilled greens and a decent Burgundy wine.

Contains protein, calcium, iron, vitamins A, B and C.

Pinto Bean Cakes

   2 tablespoons safflower oil
   1 medium onion, finely chopped
   2 cups Cooked Pinto Beans, mashed (page 44)

2 tablespoons cornmeal
½ teaspoon sea salt
1 tablespoon flour
1 teaspoon chili powder*
1 clove garlic, minced

Heat 1 tablespoon of oil and sauté onions in it for about 15 minutes, or until onions are slightly browned. Remove from heat and place in mixing bowl. Add mashed beans, cornmeal, salt, flour, and chili powder. Mix together well. If the mixture is too dry, moisten it with bean juice or a bit of water.

Heat remaining tablespoon of oil in a skillet and add garlic. Sauté until slightly browned; drop in bean mixture by the spoonful and mash each cake flat with a spatula. Brown for 5 minutes on each side, and serve. 4 to 6 cakes.

Serve from 8 months on. Just mash the cake slightly or add a bit more bean juice to moisten.

Contains protein, calcium, phosphorus, vitamins A and B.

* Omit chili powder if making cakes for children under 2 years of age.

Dinner Utamaro

2 cups Cooked Bulgur Wheat (page 44)
1 cup cooked hijiki seaweed (page 142)
5 tablespoons sunflower seeds
5 tablespoons corn oil
1 cup carrots, sliced thinly on the diagonal
1 cup broccoli or cauliflower flowerets
5 tablespoons Tamari soy sauce
5 tablespoons blackstrap molasses

In a large mixing bowl toss wheat, seaweed and seeds together lightly. Heat oil in a large wok or skillet and add carrots and broccoli or cauliflower. Sauté about 10 to 12 minutes, or until vegetables are just tender. Add soy sauce and molasses during the last two minutes of cooking. Pour carrots, broccoli and pan drippings into bowl with wheat mixture. Toss together lightly. May be eaten warm or slightly chilled. 4 servings.

Serve from 8 months on by puréeing in blender with a bit of yogurt—goat's-milk yogurt, if possible. For adults serve with chopsticks and a bottle of Japanese plum wine.

Contains protein, iron, calcium, lecithin, vitamins A, B, C, D and E.

Seaweed has long been an important food in traditional Japanese cuisine; yet only recently Americans have discovered the unique, delicious flavors of the various sea vegetables such as hijiki and nori (also called dried laver). These vegetables grow in profusion along the coasts of Japan. They are usually sun-dried to preserve the high content of trace minerals and iron. Sea vegetables are a remarkably good source of iron for a vegetarian diet.

My Best Nori Rolls (for nonbelievers)

    1½ tablespoons safflower oil
     1 large Spanish onion, chopped
    ⅔ cup pine nuts
     2 cups Steamed Brown Rice (page 42)
     1 cup cooked hijiki (page 142)
        Tamari soy sauce to taste
     8 sheets nori

Heat 1 tablespoon of oil in a skillet and add onions. Sauté over low heat until onions are very well done and nicely browned, about 20 to 25 minutes.

Heat remaining ½ tablespoon of oil and add pine nuts. Sauté slowly, stirring constantly, until nuts are browned on all sides.

In a mixing bowl combine rice, hijiki, onion, nuts and soy sauce. Spoon mixture onto sheets of nori while still warm and roll up. Let the rolls stand 1 hour before serving. They are also good served warm or cold the next day. Makes 8 rolls.

Serve from 8 months on, puréeing in the blender with ½ tablespoon Tamari soy sauce and 2 tablespoons water. These crêpelike rolls are truly delicious and make a wonderful entrée to dazzle the jaded gourmet who contends that vegetarian dinners are unsophisticated and bland. Serve them with a crisp green salad, fresh fruit compote and dry white wine.

Contains protein, iron, calcium, lecithin, vitamins A, B, C and E, as well as trace minerals.

More Nori Rolls

    2 tablespoons corn oil
    1 large Spanish onion, chopped
    ⅓ cup broccoli flowerets, cut very small
    ⅓ cup soybean sprouts
    2 tablespoons Tamari soy sauce
    2 tablespoons water
    2 cups Cooked Bulgur Wheat (page 44)
    1 cup cooked hijiki (page 142)
    8 sheets nori
       Tamari soy sauce to taste

Heat 1 tablespoon of oil in a skillet and add onions; sauté over low heat until onions are very well done and nicely browned, about 20 to 25 minutes. Remove from skillet and set aside.

Heat remaining oil in skillet and add broccoli and sprouts. Sauté over high heat for a few seconds, stirring constantly to make sure all vegetable pieces are coated with oil. After a minute or two, add Tamari soy sauce and water; reduce heat, cover and simmer slowly for a few minutes until vegetables are tender.

Combine bulgur wheat, hijiki, onions, broccoli and sprouts in a mixing bowl. Add a dash more Tamari soy sauce to suit your own taste. While still warm, spoon mixture onto sheets of nori and roll up. Let the rolls stand at least 1 hour before serving. Makes 8 rolls.

Serve from 8 months on—purée in blender with ½ tablespoon Tamari soy sauce and 2 tablespoons water.

Contains protein, iron, calcium, vitamins A, B, C, E, lecithin and trace minerals.

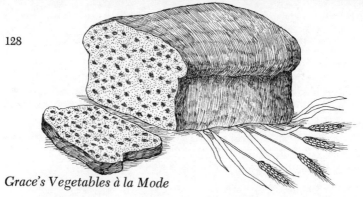

Grace's Vegetables à la Mode

    Water
1 large Spanish onion, coarsely chopped
3 medium zucchini squashes, sliced about ½ inch thick
1 pound mushrooms, sliced
⅔ cup grated Swiss cheese
1 cup yogurt

Heat about 1 inch of water to the boiling point in the bottom of a vegetable steamer; put onion in steamer and cover. Let onion steam for a few minutes and add zucchini and mushrooms; steam until vegetables are tender, about 10 minutes. Add Swiss cheese and steam until cheese begins to melt. Remove from steamer and drain of all excess liquid. Top with a cup of yogurt and serve immediately. 4 servings.

Serve from 8 months on—just purée in the blender.

Contains protein, calcium, phosphorus, vitamins A, B and C.

Spaghetti Forianno à la Ciro Cozzi

½ cup raisins
    Splash of apple juice
⅓ cup pine nuts
8 tablespoons soybean oleo (1 cube) plus 1 tablespoon
⅓ cup chopped walnuts
½ teaspoon dried basil or 4 fresh basil leaves
4 tablespoons chopped parsley
8 tablespoons safflower oil
1 clove garlic, finely minced
1 pound whole wheat spaghetti

Soak raisins in apple juice in refrigerator overnight. Drain off all excess apple juice and set raisins aside. Sauté pine nuts in 1 tablespoon oleo until browned. Combine pine nuts with raisins and walnuts and set aside. Melt rest of oleo in saucepan and add safflower oil; crush garlic in mortar with pestle, adding a tablespoon of oleo-oil combination as you grind up the garlic. Pour garlic back into saucepan and stir well. Set aside in a warm place. Cook spaghetti until tender and drain in colander. Turn out on a large warm platter and pour sauce, raisins, nuts, parsley and basil over spaghetti. Toss well with a large spoon and fork. Serve at once. 4 servings.

Serve to a child with at least 10 to 12 teeth by cutting into small pieces or puréeing in the blender with a bit of milk.

Contains iron, calcium, sodium, phosphorus, potassium, vitamins A, B, E, niacin and lecithin.

Parsley Spaghetti

- 5 tablespoons soybean oleo
- 5 tablespoons safflower oil
- 1 clove garlic, finely minced
- ½ pound whole wheat or buckwheat spaghetti
- ⅔ cup freshly grated Parmesan cheese
- ½ to ⅔ cup finely chopped parsley

Melt oleo in saucepan and add safflower oil; crush garlic in mortar with pestle, adding a tablespoon of oleo-oil combination as you crush the garlic. Pour garlic back into saucepan and stir well. Set aside in a warm place. Cook spaghetti until tender and drain in a colander. Turn out onto a large heated platter and pour oleo sauce over spaghetti. Toss well with large spoon and fork. Add cheese and toss again; add parsley and toss again. Serve at once. 2 or 3 servings.

Serve to a child with 10 to 12 teeth by cutting into small pieces.

Contains protein, calcium, lecithin, phosphorus, potassium, sodium, vitamins A, B, niacin, C and E.

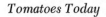

Tomatoes Today

⅔ cup Steamed Brown Rice (page 42)
⅓ cup Cooked Lentils (page 43)
2 large ripe tomatoes
⅓ cup finely minced parsley
¼ cup ground walnuts
2 teaspoons fresh or dried rosemary (ground)
2 tablespoons corn oil
Grated cheese (optional)

Cut off tops of tomatoes and scoop out insides. Mix tomato pulp with rice, lentils and remaining ingredients and stuff back into tomato shells. Sprinkle with grated cheese, if desired. Bake 15 to 20 minutes at 350° F., or until tomatoes are soft but firm. Put under broiler for a few seconds and brown tops. Serve warm. 2 servings.

Serve from 6 months on by chopping up baked tomato and combining with ½ cup yogurt and puréeing in the blender.

Contains protein, iron, lecithin, phosphorus, potassium, vitamins A, B, niacin, C and E.

Luncheon Salad

1½ cups Steamed Brown Rice, cold (page 42)
Juice of 1 lime
¼ to ⅓ cup Tamari soy sauce
¾ cup finely chopped parsley
¾ pound fresh mushrooms
Safflower oil

⅓ cup pine nuts
1 cup green beans, cut diagonally in 1-inch pieces (raw)
    Head of lettuce
    Sesame-sea salt

Toss rice with lime juice and soy sauce; add parsley and mix.
Cut mushrooms into halves or thirds, and sauté 3 to 4 minutes in
hot safflower oil; add to rice mixture. Sauté pine nuts in hot oil until
browned. Add to mixture. Sauté green beans about 4 to 7 minutes,
or until lightly browned on outside; sprinkle lightly with soy sauce
while sautéing and add to mixture. Toss all ingredients well and
allow to cool. Serve on bed of fresh lettuce, sprinkled lightly with
sesame-sea salt. 3 to 4 servings.

Serve from 6 months on—just purée in blender with a bit of
yogurt or tomato juice.

Contains protein, lecithin, phosphorus, potassium, sodium, vitamins A, C and E.

Chick-pea Salad

2 cups cooked chick-peas
¼ cup chopped pimento
½ cup chopped green pepper
½ cup celery, sliced thinly on the diagonal
6 scallions, sliced thinly on the diagonal
⅓ cup minced parsley
¾ cup mayonnaise
2 tablespoons horseradish
    Lettuce

Combine chick-peas, pimento, pepper, celery, scallions and
parsley. Toss together lightly. Combine mayonnaise and horseradish
and stir gently into salad. Arrange on a bed of crisp lettuce. 6
servings.

Serve from 1 year on by adding a bit of tomato juice and puréeing
in the blender.

Contains protein, iron, potassium, calcium, vitamins A, B and C.

Kidney Bean Salad

    2 cups cooked kidney beans
    ½ cup celery, sliced thinly on the diagonal
    ⅓ cup finely chopped dill pickles
    2 hard-boiled eggs, sliced
    4 scallions, sliced thinly on the diagonal
    ½ to ¾ cup mayonnaise
      Lettuce

Combine beans, celery, dill pickles, eggs and scallions. Toss lightly with mayonnaise and chill. Serve on a bed of crisp lettuce. 4 to 6 servings.

Serve from 1 year on by adding a little yogurt and puréeing to a coarse, choppy consistency in the blender.

Contains protein, potassium, niacin, vitamins B and C.

Garry Zimmerman's Macaroni Salad

    1 pound whole wheat macaroni
    2 cups chopped parsley
    8 scallions, sliced thinly on the diagonal
    4 hard-boiled eggs, sliced into rounds
    1½ cups cooked kidney beans
    6 celery stalks, sliced thinly on the diagonal
      Juice of one lemon
    1 cup mayonnaise
    3 tablespoons safflower oil

Cook macaroni until tender; drain and combine with remaining ingredients. 6 to 8 servings.

Serve from 10 months on by chopping coarsely in blender with a bit of yogurt to moisten.

Contains protein, lecithin, potassium, vitamins A, B, niacin and C.

EGGS

Eggs à la Ratner's Restaurant

1   Spanish onion
     Safflower oil
     Scant ½ cup water
3 or 4 fresh eggs

Chop onion coarsely (chop finely if served to small baby). Sauté in safflower oil over a low heat until wilted and softly browned, about 30 to 45 minutes. Add water, a little at a time, while sautéing, to keep onions moist. Set onions aside. Beat eggs and scramble in safflower oil. When eggs are almost done, add onions and mix lightly. 2 or 3 servings.

Serve from 7 to 8 months on. This is a good Sunday breakfast for the whole family, served with fresh orange juice and onion rolls.

Contains protein, iron, calcium, lecithin, phosphorus, potassium, sodium, vitamins A, C and E.

Snow Bird Eggs

6 eggs
    Oiled custard cups

Preheat oven to 350° F.

Separate yolks from whites of eggs. Keep each yolk separate. Beat whites with a rotary mixer or egg beater until they stand up in stiff peaks. Put whites into 6 buttered custard cups. Carefully drop a yolk into the center of each cup. Place cups in a shallow baking pan filled with about 1 inch of hot water. Bake about 5 to 7 minutes, or until whites are set.

Serve from 8 months on. This early American recipe makes a delightful breakfast or lunch treat.

Contains protein, calcium, phosphorus, iron and vitamin A.

Ox-eyes

> 6 slices whole wheat bread
> 6 eggs
>   Salt and pepper to taste
>   Bits of soybean margarine
>   Milk to cover

Preheat oven to 350° F.

Cut circles as large as possible from the slices of bread. Then cut out a smaller circle in the center of each slice. Place slices in a shallow, lightly greased baking dish. Break egg and place in the center hole of each slice. Add salt and pepper, bits of margarine and milk to cover. Bake until brown, about 30 to 45 minutes.

Serve from 6 months on. It is easily spoon-fed to a baby. This is another early American recipe.

Contains protein, calcium, phosphorus, iron and vitamin A.

Veggie Eggs Benedict

> 1 pound fresh asparagus, trimmed and steamed (page 46)
> 2 tablespoons corn oil
> 2 tablespoons grated Spanish onion
> 1 clove garlic, crushed
> 2 tablespoons whole wheat flour
> 1½ cups milk
> 1½ cups grated Cheddar cheese
> ½ teaspoon sea salt
> 6 eggs
>   Vinegar
> 6 slices whole wheat toast
>   Paprika

Drain asparagus and keep warm until serving time.

Heat oil in a heavy saucepan and add onion, garlic and flour. Add milk slowly, stirring constantly, with a wire whisk. Cook over medium heat until mixture boils. Reduce heat; add cheese and salt. Stir until cheese is completely dissolved and sauce begins to thicken. Put wax paper directly on top of the sauce to keep a skin from forming. Keep warm.

Now poach 6 eggs, using a tablespoon of vinegar for each quart of water used. Put toast on a serving dish and top with warm asparagus and a poached egg. Pour sauce over top and sprinkle with paprika. Serve at once. 6 servings.

Serve from 6 months on. A young baby can have bites of egg and sauce mixed together. This is good for a Sunday brunch entrée or for an offbeat dinner treat.

Contains protein, iron, calcium, lecithin, vitamins A, B and E.

Poached Eggs Turino

        2 large tomatoes
      ⅓ cup corn oil
        1 clove garlic, minced
            Pinch of fresh dill
        1 pound fresh spinach, washed, dried, and torn into bite-sized
              pieces
            Dash of Tamari soy sauce
        6 eggs
            Vinegar
        6 lemon wedges

Cut tomatoes into 6 slices. Heat oil in skillet and sauté garlic until slightly browned. Add tomatoes and sprinkle lightly with fresh dill. Sauté quickly on each side; remove tomato slices with a slotted spatula and drain well. To remaining hot oil add spinach and sauté for a few minutes until spinach is just barely wilted. Add soy sauce to spinach in the last few seconds of cooking, turning constantly. Heap the spinach onto a serving platter and top with tomato slices.

Meanwhile, poach 6 eggs, using a tablespoon of vinegar for every quart of water used. Place poached eggs on top of tomato slices and garnish with lemon wedges. 3 servings.

Serve this, cut up well, when a child is ready for "finger foods," at about 1 year old.

Contains protein, iron, calcium, phosphorus, lecithin, vitamins A, C and E.

VEGETABLES

Indian Eggplant Curry

      ½ teaspoon ground ginger
      ½ teaspoon ground turmeric
      1 teaspoon salt
      ¼ teaspoon chili powder
      ¼ teaspoon cinnamon
      2 tablespoons sesame seeds
      ½ cup sesame oil
      1 large eggplant, peeled and cubed
      3 large potatoes, peeled and cubed
      2 green peppers, chopped
      2 garlic cloves, crushed
   1½ cups vegetable bouillon or mixture of Tamari soy sauce and
           water
      4 tomatoes, peeled and chopped

Combine ginger, turmeric, salt, chili powder, cinnamon and sesame seeds. Set aside. Heat oil in a large skillet and add eggplant. Sauté for about 10 minutes. Dust the spices over the eggplant and turn the eggplant until it is well coated. Add potatoes, peppers, garlic and vegetable bouillon. Cover and simmer until vegetables are tender and bouillon is almost completely absorbed. Add to-

matoes and cook a few more minutes until tomatoes are tender.
4 servings.

Serve from 8 months on. Just mash slightly and add a dash of
yogurt, if desired. This is a hearty companion to any dinner entrée.

Contains calcium, lecithin, phosphorus, vitamins A, C and E.

Onion-Prune Pzazz

  1⅓ cups coarsely chopped onions
  8 to 10 large, pitted dried prunes
  ⅔ cup apple juice
  ⅓ cup water

Combine all ingredients in saucepan and bring to a boil. Cover
and lower heat. Stew slowly for 15 to 20 minutes. 3 or 4 servings.

Serve from 8 months on. To serve baby, purée in blender with
a bit of apple juice. This dish makes a good accompaniment to the
main course of a dinner.

Contains potassium, phosphorus, niacin, vitamins A and C.

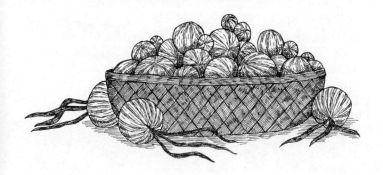

Vegetable-Nut Sauté

> 5 tablespoons vegetable oil
> 2 cups Spanish onions, coarsely chopped
> 1⅔ cup fresh green beans, sliced on the diagonal about 1 inch long
> 2 cups fresh zucchini squash, unpeeled and sliced thinly on the diagonal
> 2 cups fresh mushrooms, sliced
> 5 tablespoons Tamari soy sauce
> 1 cup almonds, unblanched and whole

Heat oil in a wok or large skillet; add onions and begin to sauté over medium heat, stirring frequently. After about 10 minutes, add green beans and continue sautéing for another 5 minutes. Add zucchini and continue for another 7 to 10 minutes. Add mushrooms and soy sauce and cook for about 2 more minutes. Add almonds and remove from heat. Let stand covered for about 10 to 15 minutes and serve. 3 to 4 servings.

Serve from 8 months on by grinding up in the blender. Use a bit of yogurt for moistening, if necessary. Serve this to the whole family for lunch or dinner with Steamed Brown Rice (page 42).

Contains protein, iron, calcium, phosphorus, lecithin, vitamins A, B, C and E.

Turkish Cucumbers

> 1 clove garlic
> 1 tablespoon lemon juice
> 2 cups yogurt
> 1½ teaspoons fresh mint, finely chopped
> 1½ teaspoons fresh dill
> 2 cucumbers

Cut garlic into small pieces and crush in mortar with pestle. Add lemon juice, mix and stir into yogurt. Chop up mint and dill finely and stir into yogurt. If fresh mint is not available, use one teaspoon of dried mint leaves, rubbed through a kitchen strainer. Peel cucumbers and cut into rounds about ⅛ inch thick. Combine with yogurt mixture and let sit in refrigerator for about 5 hours before serving. 3 or 4 servings.

Serve from 6 months on. Put ½ cup of mixture through a blender and serve for lunch or dinner vegetable.

Contains protein, calcium, phosphorus, vitamins A, B and C.

Carrot Crisp

    1 medium-size bunch carrots
      Safflower oil for sautéing
    ⅓ cup hulled sunflower seeds
    2 or 3 tablespoons Tamari soy sauce

Scrub carrots well with vegetable brush and cut into diagonal pieces. Heat oil in skillet and add carrots and seeds together. Sauté over medium flame until tender and brown, about 7 to 10 minutes. Add soy sauce while cooking. 4 servings.

Serve from 6 months on by combining ⅓ cup carrot crisp and ⅓ cup yogurt and grinding well in blender. Serve this for lunch to children with a slice of whole-grain bread spread with something like peanut or apple butter for a complete meal. Or use as a dinner vegetable.

Contains protein, iron, lecithin, potassium, vitamins A, B, C, D and E.

Christmas Sweet Potato Casserole

    1½ cups dried black mission figs
       Orange juice
     6 sweet potatoes
    ½ cup soybean oleo, melted
    ½ cup honey
     4 apples
       Nutmeg

Soak figs overnight in orange juice to cover.

Next day, wash the potatoes and cook them in boiling water for about 25 minutes, or until soft. Set aside to cool, and then peel.

In a blender combine about ⅓ cup of the orange juice in which the figs have soaked, 2 figs, oleo and honey. Pureé to a smooth sauce.

Slice the potatoes, apples and the rest of the figs. Arrange a layer of potatoes in the bottom of a casserole dish and sprinkle lightly with nutmeg. Then add a layer of figs and apples and sprinkle lightly with nutmeg. Then potatoes again and so on until all the ingredients are used up. Pour the sauce over the top of the casserole, cover and cook at 350° F. for 30 to 35 minutes. Makes 6 servings.

Serve from 8 months on—just purée in the blender. This casserole is particularily nice to serve during the holiday season.

Contains protein, calcium, iron, phosphorus, vitamins A, B and C.

Christmas Eve Beans

    5 tablespoons corn oil
    ⅓ to ½ cup pine nuts
    1 pound fresh green beans
    4 to 5 tablespoons Tamari soy sauce

Heat 1 tablespoon oil in skillet and sauté pine nuts until brown. Remove with a slotted spoon, leaving oil in skillet. Set nuts aside. Wash and cut beans diagonally. Heat oil that nuts were cooked in, adding more if necessary. Sauté beans in oil over a high heat for 7 to 10 minutes, or until still crisp, but slightly brown on the outside. Add Tamari soy sauce while cooking. Remove from heat, mix with nuts and serve. 4 servings.

Serve from 6 months on. Cut beans into small pieces and combine with nuts and a splash of tomato juice. Purée in blender to a puddinglike texture..

Contains protein, lecithin, phosphorus, potassium, vitamins A, C, E and niacin.

Extra Special Potatoes

    2 large potatoes for baking
      Safflower oil
  ½ cup yogurt
  ⅛ cup finely chopped scallions
  ⅛ cup finely chopped parsley
    1 teaspoon finely chopped fresh mint or dried mint leaves

Wash and dry potatoes; rub skins with safflower oil. Bake at 350° F. for about 1 to 1½ hours. Meanwhile, mix together remaining ingredients. If fresh mint is not available, use dried mint leaves, rubbing them in a kitchen strainer until a powdery texture is reached. Chill mixture in refrigerator. Remove potatoes from oven and split lengthwise; stuff with yogurt mixture and serve hot. 2 servings.

Serve from 4 to 6 months on. Put slightly mashed potato and yogurt mixture into blender and purée to the texture of mashed potatoes.

Contains protein, iron, calcium, phosphorus, potassium, vitamins A, B and C.

Dutch Dinner Vegetables

    2 large peeled potatoes, boiled
      Splash of milk
    2 medium peeled beets, boiled
  2½ teaspoons soybean oleomargarine
  ⅔ cup vegetable bouillon
    2 tablespoons Tamari soy sauce
      Sesame-sea salt

Mash potato until light and fluffy, adding about ¾ teaspoon margarine and a bit of milk while mashing. Set aside. Mash beets in same manner and mix together with potatoes. Combine remaining ingredients, including rest of melted margarine, and use as a sauce over the vegetables. Season with sesame-sea salt. 3 to 4 servings.

Serve from 4 months on. Use this also as a good dinner vegetable for the entire family.

Contains potassium, protein, calcium, sodium, vitamins A, B and C.

Magdalena's Dinner

       1 large Spanish onion
         Safflower oil
         Scant ½ cup water
       3 peeled potatoes, boiled
    2½ teaspoons soybean oleomargarine
         Splash of milk
       5 carrots, boiled
    ⅔ cup vegetable bouillon
       2 tablespoons Tamari soy sauce
         Sesame-sea salt

Chop onion finely and sauté in safflower oil over low heat until wilted and softly browned, about 30 to 45 minutes. Add water, a little at a time, while sautéing, to keep onions moist. Mash potatoes until light and fluffy, adding about ¾ teaspoon margarine and a splash of milk while mashing. Mash carrots with ¾ teaspoon butter until only slightly lumpy. Mix together onions, potatoes and carrots. Combine remaining ingredients, including rest of melted margarine, and use as a sauce over the vegetables. Season with sesame-sea salt. 3 to 4 servings.

Serve from 6 months on. Use this also as a good dinner vegetable for the entire family.

Contains potassium, vitamins A and C.

Hijiki Sea Vegetable

    1 cup hijiki
       Water to cover

2 tablespoons sesame oil
5 tablespoons Tamari soy sauce

Rinse hijiki thoroughly in cold water and place in a pan with water to cover. Change the water twice and then let the hijiki soak for about 15 minutes. Strain off excess water and cut into 1-inch lengths, roughly. Heat oil in a skillet and sauté the hijiki for 3 to 5 minutes, stirring constantly. Add the water used for soaking and bring to a full rolling boil. Lower flame and cover. Simmer slowly for 30 minutes. Uncover and add Tamari soy sauce. Cook over a high flame, stirring occasionally, until most of the liquid is evaporated. 2 or 3 servings.

Serve from 6 months on. Mix 1 part cooked hijiki with 2 parts cooked brown rice and purée in blender for an early basic food. It is a very good vegetable for vegetarian babies due to the high iron content. It's also good for mixing into rice salads or serving as is to the whole family.

Contains iron and iodine, all minerals and known trace minerals.

Pisto Manchego

   5 tablespoons corn oil
   1 clove garlic, finely chopped
   1 large Spanish onion, coarsely chopped
      Water to moisten
   2 large zucchini squash, sliced on the diagonal about 1½ inch
      thick
   4 large ripe tomatoes, finely chopped
   2 large potatoes, peeled and coarsely chopped
   ¾ teaspoon sea salt
   ¼ cup minced parsley
   ¼ cup Tamari soy sauce
   ½ cup water

Heat oil in a large heavy skillet; add garlic and onion and sauté until onion is completely wilted and browned, about 20 minutes.

Add a bit of water from time to time to keep the onions completely moist. Add remaining ingredients and cover skillet. Simmer slowly until vegetables are completely cooked and a rich gravy is developed, about 45 minutes. Serve hot or cold. 4 servings.

Serve from 8 months on—just purée slightly in the blender. This hearty stew makes a good dinner for the whole family.

Contains protein, calcium, iron, lecithin, phosphorus, potassium, vitamins A, B, niacin, C and E.

Zucchini Casserole

>   2 large Spanish onions
>   Safflower oil
> ¼ cup water
> ¼ cup Tamari soy sauce
>   1 large zucchini squash or 2 medium
>   1 egg, beaten
> ½ cup freshly grated Parmesan cheese

Chop onions coarsely and sauté in safflower oil about 15 to 20 minutes, or until barely wilted. Combine water and soy sauce and add gradually to cooking onions. Set aside. Cut zucchini across the width, then slice into thin strips lengthwise. Heat additional oil in skillet; dip zucchini into beaten egg and brown on both sides in oil. Drain on paper towels. In a lightly oiled casserole, put a covering of onions, then zucchini, and sprinkle with Parmesan cheese. Continue to alternate layers until vegetables are used up. Top with a dusting of Parmesan cheese and cook covered at 350° F. for 15 minutes. 4 servings.

Serve from 8 months on. To serve a baby, cut up into small pieces and run through the blender with a little tomato juice.

Contains protein, lecithin, potassium, sodium, vitamins A, B and C.

SALADS AND DRESSINGS

Agar-agar is one of the many varieties of seaweed used heavily in Oriental cuisine. Other seaweeds such as nori and hijiki are discussed on page 126. Those seaweeds are used primarily in combination with grains and vegetables or in soups. Agar-agar, however, is a gelatin and can be used in all manner of molded desserts or for fruit and vegetable aspics. Agar-agar is usually sold in bars that are about 10 to 11 inches long and 1 inch square. When softened, a bar usually makes about one cup of agar-agar. Japan is the principal source for this seaweed; you can purchase it in either health-food stores or Japanese and Chinese grocery stores.

Agar-agar Fruit Aspic

  1 bar agar-agar
  3 cups apple or cranberry juice
  6 dried apricot halves, soaked overnight in juice to cover
  ½ teaspoon cinnamon
  ½ cup fresh pineapple, chopped
  ½ cup fresh strawberries, chopped
  ⅓ cup fresh green grapes, chopped

Break the bar of agar-agar into small pieces and place in a heavy saucepan with the fruit juice; let stand about 15 to 20 minutes, or until agar-agar is softened. Meanwhile, purée the apricots in their juice in the blender until of a rich saucelike consistency. Add the apricots and cinnamon to the agar-agar and heat to the boiling point, stirring frequently; let it boil slowly for about 15 minutes, stirring frequently. Remove from heat and pour through a fine strainer to clarify the aspic and remove any undissolved particles. Let stand until lukewarm. Meanwhile, oil 6 individual molds or 1 large gelatin mold. Combine strawberries, pineapple and grapes in a mixing bowl. Pour about ⅓ inch of the agar-juice mixture into the molds and refrigerate until fairly firm. This will only take a few minutes. Meanwhile, stir the fruit into the remaining agar-juice mixture and pour it into the molds. (*If you plan to serve this aspic to an infant,* purée the pineapple, strawberries and grapes together in a blender and stir well into the agar-juice mixture. Then pour into molds.) Agar-agar molds very quickly and will often be set before it actually cools completely. To unmold, run very hot water over the outside of the mold for a few seconds and quickly invert the mold on a plate. The aspic should slide out easily; if it does stick, run more hot water over the mold. Makes 6 servings.

Serve this aspic as early as 6 months; just make sure that you purée the fruit throughly before you mix with the agar-agar. It can be introduced about the same time you start custards or yogurt. As it is, the recipe makes a very good fruit salad or dessert, particularly attractive if it's done in a well-shaped mold and garnished with orange slices and fresh cherries.

Contains iron, trace minerals, phosphorus, potassium, calcium, vitamins A, B and C.

VARIATION: Use tomato juice seasoned with a couple of teaspoons of lemon juice in place of the fruit juice and cinnamon, and use a vegetable combination such as finely chopped fresh celery and onions with steamed beets and asparagus tips to make a vegetable aspic. Unmold on a bed of watercress and garnish with lemon wedges. Serve with a very dry white wine as the first course of a special dinner.

Taboolie Salad

    3 bunches parsley
    1 cup bulgur wheat
    4 medium-size ripe tomatoes
    2 bunches scallions
    1 bunch fresh mint or dried mint leaves
    ⅓ cup safflower oil
      Juice of 3 medium-size lemons
      Juice of 1 lime

Rinse parsley thoroughly and chop up finely, discarding stems. Place in large salad bowl. Soak wheat in six cups of water for about ½ hour, or until slightly softened. Scoop wheat out of water and squeeze between palms of the hand to press out water. Toss with parsley in the bowl and set aside. Chop up tomatoes and scallions finely and toss with wheat and parsley. Chop up mint and add to salad. If dried mint is used, strain in kitchen strainer until a crude, powdery texture is achieved. Use about 2 or 3 tablespoons of mint, more if you like the minty flavor. Mix together safflower oil, lemon and lime juices and pour over salad. Toss all ingredients and let stand in refrigerator about 45 minutes to 1 hour before serving. 4 to 6 servings.

Serve from 6 months on by combining ½ cup Taboolie Salad with ⅓ cup yogurt, and purée in a blender. This traditional Lebanese dish makes a marvelous dinner salad for the whole family. Serve with a cheese omelet and hot bread.

Contains iron, calcium, lecithin, phosphorus, potassium, vitamins A, B, niacin, C and E.

Salade Bernoise

        2 cups green or red cabbage, sliced into slivers about 1½
            inches long
        2 cups Swiss cheese, sliced into slivers about 1½ inches long
        ½ cup olive oil
        ½ cup lemon juice
        4 teaspoons caraway seeds
     1½ teaspoons French mustard
        Crisp lettuce leaves

Toss cabbage and cheese together lightly. Mix oil, lemon juice, seeds and mustard thoroughly, and pour on salad. Toss lightly but thoroughly. Allow salad to marinate in the refrigerator for two hours before serving. Serve on lettuce leaves.

Serve from 1 year on. Chop in blender and use a little yogurt to moisten and sweeten for a child. This traditional French salad is good with any dinner.

Contains protein, iron, calcium, phosphorus, lecithin, vitamins A, B, C and E.

Sicilian Summer Salad

    1 avocado
    1 grapefruit
    1 pear
      Miss Ann's Special Dressing (page 154)
      Crisp lettuce
      Mint sprigs for garnish

Peel avocado and slice into sections; peel grapefruit and divide into segments. Slice pear into sections. On a bed of crisp lettuce, alternate slices of fruit. Garnish with sprigs of mint and pour dressing over fruit. Serve immediately. 3 or 4 servings.

Serve from 6 months on. Just put avocado, grapefruit, and pear slices in blender with a bit of dressing. Purée to a puddinglike texture.

Contains potassium, vitamins A and C.

Miss Ann's Midwinter Salad

    ½ cup raisins
       Apple juice
    1 large apple
    ⅓ to ½ cup yogurt

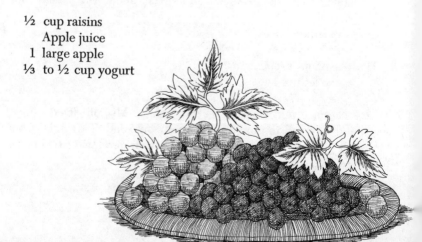

1 teaspoon honey
2 cups grated carrots
  Crisp lettuce

Soak raisins overnight in apple juice in refrigerator. Core apple but leave unpeeled. Dice into small pieces and combine with yogurt and honey. Purée to the consistency of mayonnaise. In a bowl combine carrots and raisins. (Drain raisins of excess juice.) Mix with yogurt dressing and serve on a bed of crisp lettuce. 3 or 4 servings.

Serve from 6 months on. Just purée dressing, carrots and raisins together in blender. Very good for a baby.

Contains calcium, protein, phosphorus, potassium, vitamins A, B and C.

Special Spinach Bowl

1 pound raw spinach
3 medium tomatoes
½ pound fresh mushrooms
  Safflower oil for sautéing
1 clove garlic, minced
  Tamari soy sauce
  Basic Dressing (page 153)
2 hard-boiled eggs

Wash and dry all vegetables thoroughly. Tear spinach into bite-size pieces and put in salad bowl. Cut up tomatoes and add to spinach. Cut mushrooms into halves or thirds. Heat oil in skillet and add garlic. Sauté until garlic is slightly brown; then add mushrooms and sauté for a minute or two. Sprinkle lightly with soy sauce and stir well in skillet. Remove to plate to cool. Add to salad and toss well. Add dressing and toss again. Slice eggs thinly into rounds and add to salad. Toss lightly. 4 servings.

Serve from 1 year on or when baby has 10 to 12 teeth and can chew well. This salad makes a good dinner accompaniment or complete luncheon served with rye crackers and sliced cheese.

Contains calcium, lecithin, potassium, sodium, niacin, vitamins A, B, C and E.

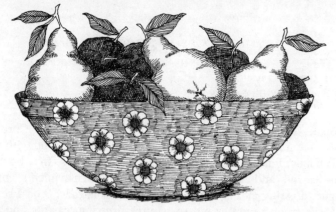

Simple Simon's Salad

1 medium head butter lettuce
1 small bunch watercress
6 scallions
3 heaping tablespoons parsley, finely minced
Basic Dressing (page 153)

Wash all vegetables thoroughly and drain of all excess water. Tear lettuce into bite-size pieces and put into a salad bowl. Chop up watercress into small pieces and add to lettuce. Slice scallions very thinly on the diagonal and add to salad, along with parsley. Toss all ingredients together and add dressing. Toss again. 4 servings.

Serve from 1 year on, or from when baby has 10 to 12 teeth. Cut into small pieces.

Contains potassium, vitamins A, C and E; also iron, lecithin phosphorus and protein.

Mr. Gilhooley's Salad

4 tangerines
1 Spanish onion
Miss Ann's Special Dressing (page 154)
Fresh mint sprigs
Crisp lettuce

Peel tangerines and separate into individual segments. Slice onion into thin rings and cut rings in half. Mix together with tangerine segments and marinate in dressing. Allow to marinate about 2 or 3 hours before serving. Arrange on a bed of crisp lettuce and garnish with sprigs of fresh mint. 4 servings.

Serve from 1 year on.

Contains calcium, lecithin, potassium, vitamins A, C and E.

Vegetable Dip

¼ cup sour cream
3 tablespoons tomato soup
1 tablespoon finely grated onion
1 teaspoon sea salt
1 tablespoon finely chopped parsley
  Sea salt to taste

Combine all ingredients and serve surrounded by cauliflower flowerets, celery stalks, carrot slices and cherry tomatoes.

Serve from 1 year on (or whenever baby has enough teeth to begin chewing on the crisper fresh vegetables).

Contains protein, iron, calcium, phosphorus, vitamins A, B and C.

Grace Fass's Good Dressing

½ teaspoon celery seed
½ cup raw sugar
1½ teaspoons dry mustard
1½ teaspoons sea salt
¼ cup vinegar
1½ tablespoons grated onion
1 cup corn or safflower oil

Mix together all ingredients but the oil. Pour into a blender and stir for about 7 to 10 minutes, adding the oil very slowly. Serve this dressing over a combination salad of avocados, oranges and walnuts, or over fresh beets.

Serve from 2 years on.

Contains calcium, lecithin, phosphorus, vitamins A, B, C and E.

Grace's Grandma's Green Goddess Dressing

    2 tablespoons finely chopped scallions
    1 clove garlic, crushed
    ¼ cup finely chopped parsley
    1 cup mayonnaise
    ½ cup sour cream or yogurt
    1 tablespoon lemon juice
    ¼ cup vinegar
    ¼ cup crumbled Roquefort cheese
       Sea salt and pepper to taste

Combine all ingredients and let sit in refrigerator for 2 days before serving.

Serve over cold, crisp greens. Serve from 1 year on.

Contains protein, iron, calcium, phosphorus, vitamins A, B and C.

Never-failing Mayonnaise
(early American style)

    1 tablespoon mashed potato
    ¼ teaspoon sea salt
       Yolk of one egg, beaten
    ¾ cup olive oil
       Pepper and paprika to taste
    2 teaspoons vinegar

Combine potato, salt and egg. Add the olive oil slowly, stirring with a wire whisk at each addition. Then add vinegar and season with pepper and paprika to taste. More oil and vinegar may be added if a larger quantity is needed.

Use with any salad as a dressing. When children are ready for "finger foods" and you want to introduce them to raw vegetables, use this mayonnaise as a dip. Cut carrots, celery, etc., into sticks and let your child dip them into the mayonnaise.

Contains protein, calcium, iron, lecithin, phosphorus, vitamins A, C and E.

Your Own Very Quick Mayonnaise

  1 egg
  2 teaspoons lemon juice
  ½ teaspoon sea salt
  1 teaspoon powdered kelp
  1 teaspoon honey
  1 teaspoon paprika
  1 clove garlic, cut up
  1 cup safflower oil

Combine egg, lemon juice, salt, kelp, honey, paprika, garlic and
¼ cup oil in blender. Purée about 15 seconds on slow speed while
adding remaining oil at a fast, steady pace. Oil must be mixed in
by the end of the 15 seconds. Blend 3 more seconds at highest speed.
Serve from 6 months on with all salads calling for mayonnaise.

Contains protein, calcium, iron, lecithin, vitamins A, C and E.

Basic Dressing

  1 clove garlic
  ½ cup vegetable oil (safflower, corn, sesame, avocado, etc.)
  ½ cup lemon or lime juice

Mince garlic and crush in mortar with pestle. Add a little oil and
grind together. When garlic is thoroughly crushed and absorbed into
oil, mix together with remaining oil and the juice.
Serve from 9 months.

Contains lecithin and vitamins A, C and E.

A Dressing for Fruit Desserts

  ½ cup yogurt
  ½ cup sour cream
  2 teaspoons buckwheat honey
 10 to 12 ripe strawberries
  ½ a ripe banana

Purée all ingredients in blender to the consistency of a rich mayonnaise. Mix with any fresh fruit such as blueberries, strawberries, chopped apples with nuts, etc. Use any combination that pleases you; just stick to the fresh fruits that are currently in season in your own area. 4 servings.

Serve from 6 months on. Purée with fruit for baby's dessert.

Contains protein, calcium, iron, phosphorus, potassium, vitamins A, B and C.

Miss Ann's Special Dressing

- ¾ cup safflower oil
- ¼ cup fresh lime juice
- ⅛ cup fresh lemon juice
- 2 teaspoons honey
- 1 small clove garlic, minced and slightly crushed
- 1 teaspoon sea salt
- 2 teaspoons finely minced mint leaves
- ¼ teaspoon freshly ground white peppercorns

Combine all ingredients in refrigerator jar; cover and shake well to blend all ingredients thoroughly.

Serve from 1 year on.

Contains lecithin, potassium, vitamins A, C and E.

SOUPS

With the exception of those that contain yogurt, nearly every soup (or other combination foods such as sauces or casseroles) is better the second day. The time lapse allows for a subtle blending and deepening of the combined flavors. It gains a certain richness that only time will permit. If you do serve soup the same day it is prepared, allow it to stand at least an hour after the cooking time. Serve soup "very warm" and never "piping hot," as intense heat causes a loss in the delicacy of the flavors. This rule is well observed with all hot foods, as the body more easily assimilates foods taken in at lower temperatures.

Chilled Cranberry Soup

    1 pound fresh cranberries
1½ cups honey
    1 cup water
    1 cup apple juice
    1 orange
   ½ lemon
    1 cup yogurt
    1 ripe banana

Combine cranberries, honey, water and apple juice in large saucepan. Peel orange and divide into segments. Cut segments into thirds and add to cranberries. Slice lemon into very thin rounds; halve the lemon rounds and add to cranberries. Bring mixture to a boil over a medium flame and then boil very rapidly for about 3 to 5 minutes, or until cranberries begin to pop. Remove from heat, cover and let cool.

Purée cranberry mixture in blender until frothy. Set aside. Purée yogurt and banana until a milkshake consistency is reached. Stir yogurt-banana mixture into cranberry purée and chill well before serving. Garnish with thin slices of lime cut into rounds. 6 to 8 servings.

Serve from 6 months on. This makes a wonderful appetizer for a summer dinner party. To serve a baby, mix with equal parts of milk and serve in a bottle. You can also serve as is and spoon-feed.

Contains protein, calcium, phosphorus, potassium, vitamins A, B and C.

Eva Moroian's Yogurt Soup

    1 cup barley
    4 cups water
    1 egg
    2 cups yogurt
   ⅛ pound soybean oleo (optional)

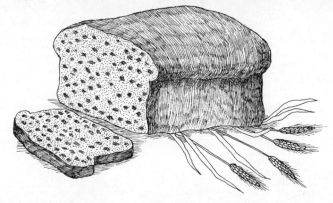

Soak barley overnight in water. Bring it to a boil in the same water and let simmer about 45 minutes. Beat egg into the yogurt and pour it gradually into the cooking barley. Stir constantly to avoid curdling the yogurt. Bring to a boil, stirring constantly. Immediately remove from the heat and add about ⅛ pound soybean oleo if you are serving it hot. To serve chilled, leave out the oleo and chill. Garnish hot soup with paprika and minced parsley, and cold soup with lemon rounds. 4 to 6 servings.

Serve from 4 to 6 months on. Just purée a few seconds in the blender to dissolve the barley. It can be spoon-fed or put in a bottle with an enlarged opening in the nipple.

Contains protein, calcium, phosphorus, potassium, sodium, vitamins A and B.

Mrs. Moroian's Noodle Soup

    ½ to 1 cup lentils
    1 or 2 cups water
    ⅛ pound soybean oleo
    1 cup noodles
    1 egg
    2 cups yogurt

Boil lentils in water for about ½ hour. Drain and set aside. Break noodles into small pieces and brown slowly in the oleo. When noodles are nicely browned, add 2 cups water and cook until noodles are done, about 15 minutes. Beat egg into yogurt and pour gradually into noodles, stirring constantly. Add lentils and remove from heat. Vary consistency of the soup with water. Serve warm. 4 servings.

Serve from 4 to 6 months on. Just purée in blender until lentils and noodles are dissolved. Spoon-feed or use bottle with enlarged nipple opening.

Contains protein, calcium, iron, phosphorus, potassium, sodium, vitamins A and B.

Bengalese Lentil Soup
(exotic and darkly delicious)

    6 cups vegetable bouillon*
    1 cup lentils
    1 large potato, unpeeled and coarsely chopped
    2 tablespoons safflower or corn oil
    1 large Spanish onion, chopped
    2 tomatoes, peeled, seeded and finely chopped†
    1 teaspoon caraway seeds
    1 dill pickle, finely chopped
      Juice of ½ lemon
      Sea salt and pepper to taste

In a soup kettle bring 6 cups of vegetable bouillon to a boil and add the lentils. Cover and simmer slowly for about 1 hour, or until lentils are tender. Then add the potatoes and continue to simmer.

Meanwhile, heat the oil in a skillet and sauté the onions until tender, about 10 minutes. Add the tomatoes and caraway seeds and cook together for about 3 minutes.

Add onion-tomato mixture, dill pickle, and lemon juice to the soup kettle. Continue to simmer for 1 to 1½ hours. Season with salt and pepper to taste during the last hour of cooking. 4 to 6 servings.

Serve from 8 months on. Purée to a creamy texture in the blender. This hearty soup, together with any fruit salad, Christmas Eve Beans (page 140), and hot rolls makes a very substantial dinner.

Contains protein, calcium, iron, phosphorus, potassium, vitamins A, B and C.

---

* Most gourmet or organic specialty food stores carry vegetable bouillon cubes. The vegetable bouillon imported from Switzerland is the most flavorful.
† Plunge tomatoes into boiling water for a minute or two; remove, cool, and skins will peel off with ease.

Pistachio-Lentil Soup . . . so good!

>   2 tablespoons safflower oil
> 1½ cups Spanish onion, chopped medium fine
>   1 cup carrots, coarsely chopped
>   7 or 8 cups vegetable bouillon (cubes may be used) (use 7
>   cups for a thicker soup)
> 1½ cups lentils
>   2 tablespoons tomato paste
>   ½ teaspoon ground cumin seed
>   ⅛ teaspoon turmeric
>   ¾ cup pistachio nuts, skinned* and coarsely chopped
>   Sea salt and pepper to taste

In a skillet heat the oil and add the onion and carrots; sauté until onion is transparent, about 7 or 8 minutes.

Heat the vegetable bouillon; add onions, carrots, lentils, tomato paste and seasonings. Bring to a boil and cover; reduce the heat and simmer very slowly for 2½ to 3 hours. Put the soup through a sieve and return to the soup kettle. Add pistachio nuts, salt and pepper, and reheat. 6 servings.

Serve from 8 months on. Just purée the soup in a blender to crush the nuts for baby. This very tasty soup, based in part on a Turkish folk recipe, makes a good winter dinner served with a salad of crisp greens, and spinach noodles lightly tossed with butter and Parmesan cheese. Crown your meal with a hearty Burgundy.

Contains protein, calcium, phosphorus, potassium, sodium, vitamins A, B and C.

---

* Plunge pistachios into boiling water for a few minutes. Drain, let cool and the skins will peel off easily.

Vegetable Soup

>   4 medium carrots, sliced on the diagonal into 1-inch pieces
>   1 medium-size turnip, chopped into bite-size pieces

 1 medium-size Spanish onion, chopped coarsely
 3 vegetable bouillon cubes
 6 cups water
   Handful of egg noodles
 3 tablespoons chopped parsley
1½ cups sliced fresh mushrooms
1½ teaspoons Tamari soy sauce (optional)

Combine carrots, turnip, onion, bouillon cubes and water in a covered kettle. Heat and let simmer about 20 to 25 minutes. Add noodles and cook another 10 minutes. Add parsley and mushrooms and cook another 10 minutes. Stir in soy sauce just before serving, if desired. 4 to 6 servings.

Serve from 4 to 6 months on. Just whirl for a few seconds in the blender to purée the vegetables and noodles. The soup can be spoon-fed or put in a bottle with an enlarged nipple opening.

Contains protein, iron, calcium, phosphorus, potassium, sodium, vitamins A, niacin and C.

DESSERTS

Prune Whip

 1 pound prunes
 2 tablespoons honey plus honey for garnish
   Whites of 6 eggs
   Yogurt

Soak prunes overnight in water to cover. In the morning, bring prunes to a boil, cover and let simmer slowly until prunes are soft, about 30 to 40 minutes. Add 2 tablespoons honey as they cook. Remove from heat and drain. Remove the stones from the prunes and purée to a paste in the blender. Beat egg whites with a rotary mixer or egg beater until they stand in stiff peaks. Fold whites in prune paste and turn into a buttered baking dish. Bake about 20 to 25 minutes at 300° F. Serve cold, garnished with a dash of yogurt and honey. 4 to 6 servings.

Serve from 6 months on.

Contains protein, iron, calcium, phosphorus, vitamins A and C.

Banana Bonanza

    2 large medium-ripe bananas
    ½ cup sifted whole wheat flour
       Soybean oleomargarine for sautéing
    ½ cup chopped walnuts
       Honey

Peel bananas and cut in half lengthwise and then cut again crosswise. Sprinkle with flour and sauté in margarine until lightly browned. Drain on paper towels and place on a warm platter. Dot with honey and sprinkle with nuts. Serve at once. 4 servings.

Serve from 8 months on—just mash slightly and omit the nuts.

Contains potassium, protein, vitamin A.

> There was an old woman lived under the hill,
> And if she's not gone she lives there still.
> Baked apples she sold, and cranberry pies,
> And she's the old woman that never told lies.
> —MOTHER GOOSE

Baked Apple Dessert

    4 dried apricots
    ½ cup raisins
       Apple juice to cover
    4 whole apples
    ⅛ to ¼ cup crushed hazelnuts
    ½ cup honey mixed with ½ cup hot water

Chop apricots into small pieces and combine with raisins; soften overnight in refrigerator with apple juice to cover. Take sharp-edged spoon, knife, or corer and hollow out center of apples. Stuff apples tightly with mixture of raisins, apricots, the soaking juice and the nuts. Place in a shallow baking pan and cover with honey water mixture. Bake at 350° F., basting occasionally with residue juices until done, about 45 minutes. Serve warm. 4 servings.

Serve from 6 months on. To serve a baby, let apple cool and scoop out stuffing and apple pulp. Combine in blender with ½ cup yogurt and some of the cooking juices and purée to a pudding consistency.

Contains phosphorus, potassium, vitamins A, B, C and E.

Apple Flip

 ¼ to ⅓ cup raisins
  Apple juice to cover
 2 apples
  Safflower oil
  Cinnamon

Soften raisins in apple juice overnight in refrigerator; slice un-peeled but cored apples into crescent shapes and sauté in safflower oil until soft. Add cinnamon to taste while sautéing; mix in raisins and apple juice when nearly done. Serve warm. 4 servings.

Serve from 6 months on. To serve a baby, let mixture cool after cooking, place in blender with a bit of apple juice and purée a few seconds.

Contains phosphorus, potassium, vitamins A, C and E.

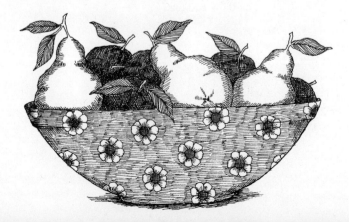

Dappled Apples

    5 large firm apples
    1 cup Vermont maple syrup
  ¼ teaspoon cinnamon
  ¼ teaspoon nutmeg
  ½ cup browned and buttered bread crumbs
  ½ cup currants
    2 teaspoons grated lemon rind
    4 slices whole wheat bread

Peel, core and cut apples into small chunks. Combine with maple syrup, cinnamon and nutmeg and cook over a low heat until barely cooked. Drain the apples and save the syrup. Spread the bread crumbs over the bottom of a 9-inch casserole and sprinkle with a few currants. Add apples, remaining currants and sprinkle with lemon rind. Trim crusts from bread and butter both sides of slices. Cut into triangles and place on top of apples. Spoon reserved syrup over the bread, making sure it saturates entire casserole. Bake 15 minutes at 400° F., or until the bread is browned.

Serve from 9 months on—just mash very well. 4 servings.

Contains phosphorus, potassium, vitamins A, C and E.

> Pat-a-cake, pat-a-cake,
> Baker's Man!
> So I do, master, as fast as I can.
> Pat it, and prick it
> And mark it with B
> And then it will serve
> For Baby and me.
> —MOTHER GOOSE

Abby's Carrot Cake

    2 cups whole wheat flour
    2 cups raw sugar
    2 teaspoons baking soda

    2 teaspoons sea salt
    2 teaspoons cinnamon
1½ cups safflower oil
    4 eggs
    3 cups grated carrots, tightly packed

Preheat oven to 350° F. Mix together dry ingredients and sift
together twice. Add oil and stir well. Add eggs, one at a time, and
mix well with each addition. Add carrots and stir well. Bake in 3
standard cake pans (loaf, square or round), greased and lightly
floured. Bake for 25 to 30 minutes. Turn out onto a cake rack and
let cool for at least 20 minutes before serving.

Serve from 6 months on. This makes a very moist, delicious cake.
Serve it with a bit of cream or yogurt to young babies. This is
another good party cake.

Contains protein, phosphorus, potassium, vitamins A, B and C.

Orange Blossom Cake

    1 cup honey
    2 tablespoons safflower oil
    1 egg, well beaten
    1 tablespoon grated orange rind
½ tablespoon grated lemon rind
2½ cups sifted whole wheat flour
2½ teaspoons baking powder
½ teaspoon baking soda
½ teaspoon sea salt
¾ cup fresh orange juice
¾ cup chopped walnuts

Preheat oven to 325° F. Combine honey and oil and mix together
well; add egg and orange and lemon rinds. Sift together all dry ingredients and add to the honey-oil mixture, a little at a time, alternating with the orange juice. Stir until just mixed. Mix the nuts in
and bake in a greased, lightly floured 9-inch loaf pan at 325° F.
for 1 hour and 10 minutes.

Serve from 8 months on. This is also very good toasted and spread with cream cheese.

Contains protein, lecithin, phosphorus, vitamins A, B and C.

Sara Charnis' Special Cake
(Molasses and Dried Apple Cake)

- 2 cups dried apples
- 1 cup crude molasses
- ⅔ cup sweet butter
- 1 cup raw sugar
- 1 cup milk
- 2 eggs, well beaten
- 1 cup raisins
- 2 cups whole wheat flour
- 1 cup unbleached white flour
- 2 teaspoons baking powder
- 1 teaspoon soda
- 1 teaspoon cinnamon
- 1 teaspoon nutmeg

Preheat oven to 325° F.

Place apples in a blender and chop them up. In a heavy saucepan, simmer apples and molasses together for about 15 minutes. Let cool.

With a rotary mixer or egg beater, cream butter and sugar together. Add milk slowly, beating constantly; add beaten eggs and beat again. With a spoon, stir in raisins and the apple-molasses mixture.

Sift together all dry ingredients and add to the apple-molasses mixture. Mix together thoroughly.

Grease and lightly flour a 9 x 3½-inch spring-form pan. Turn cake into pan and bake for about 1 hour, or until a toothpick inserted in the center comes out clean.

Serve from 8 months on. This makes a delicious, rich, heavily textured cake.

Contains protein, calcium, phosphorus, iron, lecithin, vitamins A, B and C.

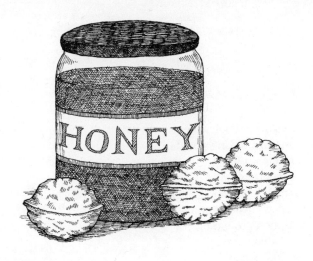

Christmas Fruit Cake

- 1 cup pitted dates
- 1 cup dried figs
- 1 cup sunflower seeds
- 1 cup shredded coconut, unsweetened
- 1 cup raisins
- 1 cup almonds
- 1 cup walnuts
- 1 orange, peeled
   Juice of 1 orange
   Juice of 1 lemon
   Juice of 2 apples
- 1 cup Vermont maple syrup
- 1 cup currants
- 1 teaspoon cinnamon
- ½ teaspoon nutmeg

In a food chopper grind dates, figs, sunflower seeds, coconut, raisins, almonds, walnuts and peeled orange. Add remaining ingredients and work together well. Pack solidly in a loaf pan and let harden in refrigerator.

Serve from 9 months on.

Contains protein, iron, potassium, phosphorus, vitamins A, C and D.

Gingerbread

- 1 tablespoon apple-cider vinegar
- ¾ cup milk
- 2 cups sifted whole wheat flour
- 2 teaspoons baking powder
- ¼ teaspoon soda
- ½ teaspoon salt
- 2 teaspoons ground ginger
- 1 teaspoon ground cinnamon
- ¼ teaspoon ground cloves
- ⅓ cup safflower oil
- ½ cup raw sugar
- 1 egg
- ¾ cup molasses

Preheat oven to 350° F.

Add vinegar to milk and set aside. Combine flour, baking powder, soda, salt, and spices; sift together twice. Cream the sugar and safflower oil together; add the egg and beat until light and fluffy. Add molasses and stir well. Add dry ingredients, a little at a time, alternating with milk, which should be curdled at this point. After each addition, stir only until just mixed.

Bake in an 8 x 8 x 2-inch pan, lightly greased and floured, for about 45 to 50 minutes. To test, press gently in the center; if bread rises after your touch, it's done.

Serve from 9 months on.

Contains protein, calcium, sodium, phosphorus, potassium, niacin and lecithin.

Charlie Wag ate the pudding and left the bag
Sing, sing, what shall I sing?
The cat ran away with the pudding bag string.
            —MOTHER GOOSE

Indian Pudding

1½ cups small California currants
 3 cups scalded milk
1½ cups cold milk
 1 cup cornmeal
 ½ cup blackstrap molasses
 ½ cup buckwheat honey
 1 teaspoon salt
 ¾ teaspoon ginger
 ¼ teaspoon nutmeg
 ¼ cup safflower oil

Combine currants and hot milk; set aside. Stir 1 cup cold milk
into cornmeal and add to the hot-milk mixture. Heat on a very low
flame, stirring constantly until mixture thickens, about 15 minutes.
Add molasses, honey, salt, ginger, nutmeg and oil. Pour into a
buttered 2-quart casserole and pour the remaining ½ cup cold milk
into the center of the pudding. Set dish in a pan of cold water and
bake for 2½ hours at 300° F. Let cool at least 3 hours before
serving. 4 to 6 servings.
   Serve from 6 months. Just purée slightly to break up the currants.

Contains protein, calcium, iron, niacin, potassium, vitamins A
and C.

Brown Rice Pudding

 4 cups goat's milk
 ⅔ cup buckwheat honey
 ¼ cup uncooked brown rice

½ teaspoon salt
1 teaspoon vanilla
   Freshly grated nutmeg
½ cup dried figs, finely chopped
2 eggs, well beaten

Combine milk, honey, rice, salt and vanilla. Put in a casserole and grate a little fresh nutmeg over the top. Bake uncovered, at 300° F. for 3 hours. During the first hour stir 3 or 4 times so the rice won't settle on the bottom of the dish. After the first hour, stir in the figs. After 2½ hours, stir in the eggs. 4 to 6 servings.

Serve from 6 months on. You may want to run it through the blender a few seconds for younger babies. This is a very good dessert for the whole family.

Contains protein, calcium, iron, potassium, vitamins A and B.

Baby Custard

6 egg yolks
½ cup honey
¼ teaspoon salt
3 cups scalded milk
1 teaspoon vanilla
   nutmeg

Beat egg yolks just enough to blend them together evenly; stir in honey and salt. Add milk and vanilla, a little at a time; beat continually with a fork. Pour into 6 buttered custard cups and sprinkle with nutmeg. Set cups in shallow pan on a paper towel. Add about an inch of hot water. Bake for 45 minutes at 350° F. Test by inserting a silver knife near the edge of the custard; if it comes out clean, custard is done. Let cool before serving. 6 servings.

Serve from 6 months on. A wonderful treat for baby; serve often. Also good for pregnant women.

Contains protein, calcium, lecithin, phosphorus, potassium, vitamins A, B and C.

Cranberry Sauce for Pancakes or French Toast

>   2 apples, unpeeled
>   1 pound fresh cranberries
> 1½ cups apple cider
>   1 cup honey

Chop apples and put in blender with enough cider to facilitate blending. Blend until apples are a smooth, liquidy consistency. Combine apples with rest of ingredients in a saucepan and heat to the boiling point. Reduce heat slightly and continue to cook until berries pop, about 5 to 8 minutes. Cover and let cool. Pour about half of the mixture into the blender and purée until creamy smooth. Combine with remaining solid berries and use as a syrup on pancakes, French toast, ice cream or any other dish calling for syrup. Makes about 1 quart.

Serve from 6 months on.

Contains calcium, phosphorus, vitamins A, B and C.

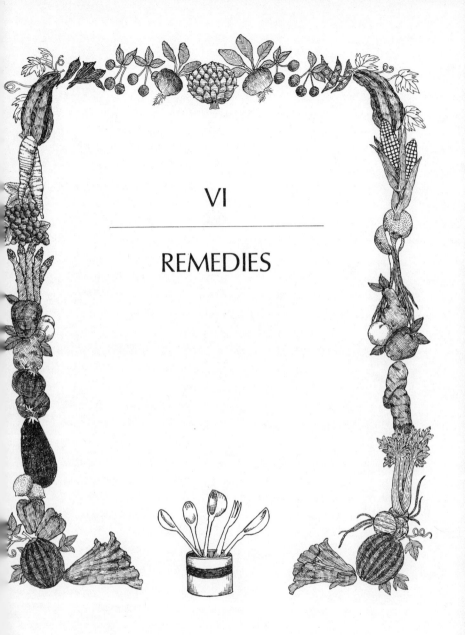

VI

REMEDIES

Rainy Day and Runny Nose Lunch

    2 whole oranges, unpeeled
    2 apples, peeled and cored
    ½ cup apple cider
    ½ cup water
    4 tablespoons honey
       Freshly grated nutmeg
       Liquid vitamin C
       Ground walnuts (optional)

Slice oranges into very thin rounds and quarter them; dice apples and combine with oranges in saucepan. Pour in cider, water and honey; mix together. Add nutmeg. Heat to boiling point; reduce heat and cover. Let simmer about 10 to 15 minutes. Remove from heat and let cool in covered pan. Purée in blender to the consistency of apple sauce. Add a level teaspoonful of liquid vitamin C to each serving. Use a teaspoonful of nuts per serving, if desired.

Serve from 6 months on. Serve for lunch and dinner when baby's cold is bad. Or fill a bottle about ⅓ full with mixture and add ⅔ bottle apple juice. Give to baby at bedtime.

Contains calcium, potassium, niacin, vitamins A and C.

The Winter Cold Special

> 1 pound fresh cranberries, washed and sorted
> 1 cup water
> ½ cup fresh orange juice
> ½ cup apple juice
> 1½ cups honey
> 1 lemon, sliced thinly into rounds, then halved
> 1 grapefruit, peeled and separated into segments
> Freshly grated nutmeg
> Liquid vitamin C

Combine cranberries with water, orange juice, apple juice and honey; add lemon rounds. Cut grapefruit segments into thirds and add to cranberries. Grate in nutmeg and bring to a boil. Let simmer a few minutes until berries begin to pop. Turn off heat and let stand, covered, until cool. Purée in blender until light and frothy. Serve as is, or dilute ½ to ⅓ with water in the baby's bottle. Add an even teaspoon of liquid vitamin C to each bottleful. Also use this over cereal in place of milk or yogurt. Makes about 2 quarts.

Serve from 6 months on whenever baby has a cold. Can be used in place of milk until runny nose ceases. Avoid dairy products such as yogurt and cottage cheese, as these are mucus-forming foods.

Contains potassium, vitamins A, B_1 and C.

Sleet and Snow Supper

> 1 apple, peeled, cored and diced
> ½ lemon, sliced into thin rounds and quartered
> 1 cup fresh orange juice
> ⅓ cup water
> 2 tablespoons honey
> ¾ cup acorn squash, baked
> Freshly grated nutmeg
> Cinnamon
> Liquid vitamin C

Combine apple, lemon, orange juice, water and honey in saucepan. Grate in nutmeg. Bring to a boil, reduce heat, and cover. Cook for 3 minutes. Let cool in covered pan. Purée in blender to the consistency of applesauce. Add squash and cinnamon and purée again. Add a level teaspoon of liquid vitamin C to every serving. 2 servings.

Serve from 6 months on. This makes a very good lunch or dinner whenever baby has a bad cold, as it is free of mucus-producing dairy products and has a high vitamin C content.

Contains iron, potassium, vitamins A and C.

Dinner for a Constipated Baby

2 dried prunes
2 dried apricots
  Prune juice
1 tablespoon cream cheese
2 tablespoons yogurt

Soak prunes and apricots overnight in prune juice to cover; pour into blender and purée. Add cheese and yogurt and purée again. 1 or 2 servings.

Serve from 6 months on for breakfast or lunch.

Contains protein, calcium, iron, potassium, sodium, niacin, vitamins A, B and C.

Early American Cough Medicine

3 tablespoons lemon juice
3 tablespoons olive oil
3 tablespoons honey

Mix thoroughly and feed 1 teaspoonful at a time to a coughing child. Can be given every 2 or 3 hours.

Serve from 6 months on.

Contains calcium, phosphorus, lecithin, vitamins C and E.

Diaper Rash Remedy

Safflower oil
Cornstarch

When your baby develops a diaper rash, rub his whole bottom-side throughly with safflower oil and then powder it with cornstarch. During the day, leave off the diaper as much as possible, as exposure to the air promotes rapid healing.

Crusty-Behind-the-Ears Remedy

Safflower oil

At one time or another, babies get a kind of scabby crust behind their ears. Rub the back of the ears thoroughly with safflower oil and the condition should clear up in a couple of days.

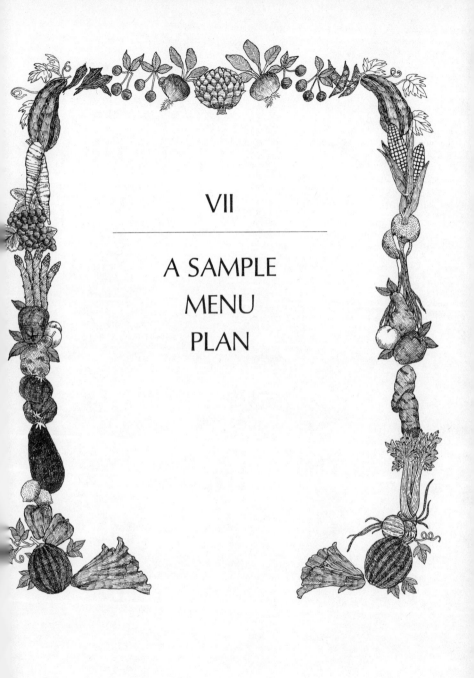

VII

A SAMPLE
MENU
PLAN

This is a sample menu plan for a period covering one week. I have stayed within the traditional three-meals-a-day format. You may find, however, that your child has made up a completely new schedule for himself. My own son has never taken more than two full meals a day, and he preferred to do most of his eating during the morning, while eating very lightly in the evening. During the warm summer months, especially, he was not inclined to accept much food around noonday, and seemed to favor fruit drinks (see Chapter IV) in the afternoon.

I have used one basic formula throughout the menu plan for a bedtime drink. The Basic Formula (page 89) contains milk, yeast and banana. I gave this to my son every night. Yeast is very important in the diet of a vegetarian baby as it contains high amounts of protein, iron and amino acids. In the recipe I used the ratio of ingredients that my own son adapted to easily. I suggest consulting your own pediatrician about the exact amounts of yeast suitable for your baby at various stages of development. I started with a teaspoon of yeast when he was six months old and worked up to a heaping tablespoon of yeast by the time he was one year old.

I think it's best not to force a child to eat. Children seem to know intuitively what's best for them in this regard. As long as your child is maintaining an adequate weight gain, I don't think you have to be too concerned. Just keep in touch with a medical authority that you trust, especially during the first year of life. After that it's all easier, because your baby is bigger, heartier, and you know him much better.

Sometime between a year and two years old (roughly) most children go through a phase where they barely eat anything at all and often reject foods that they previously loved. This can really drive a mother crazy with worry and fears that the child cannot sustain himself. But as a doctor friend of mine said, it's common knowledge that two-year-olds live on air. Just remember that no child ever starved where food was available. During this phase, particularly, it's very tempting to try to force food upon your baby. But that is virtually impossible anyway, and it only angers and frustrates the child. Be patient and he will eat well again, though it may take months. What you can do is add a tablespoon of yeast to his naptime bottle in addition to the one tablespoon already given in the nighttime bottle. Also look at Chapter IV for ideas on what extras you can put in his drinks because a child never quits drinking even though he may be eating poorly.

Sunday

BREAKFAST
Abigail Van Derek's Incredible Granola (page 32). Contains grains, nuts, fruits. Serve with milk or yogurt and a banana.

LUNCH
Blue Plate Special (page 76). Contains bulgur wheat, squash, yogurt.

DINNER
Burgie Delight or Soyball Sensation (page 111). Contains soybeans, onions, cheese, peanuts. Serve with *Baked Apple Dessert* (page 160). Contains apples, raisins, apricots, nuts.

BEDTIME
The Basic Formula (page 89). Contains yeast, milk, banana.

Monday

BREAKFAST
Soy Pancakes (page 52). Contains soybeans, egg, milk. Serve with *Cranberry Sauce* (page 169). Contains cranberries, apples, honey.

LUNCH

Baby's Mexican Dinner (page 79). Contains tomato, avocado, cottage cheese and yogurt.

DINNER

Lentil Loaf à la Damascus (page 116). Contains lentils, cheese, onions, whole wheat bread crumbs. Serve with *Christmas Sweet Potato Casserole* (page 139). Contains sweet potatoes, apples, figs, orange.

BEDTIME

The Basic Formula (page 89). Contains yeast, milk, banana.

Tuesday

BREAKFAST

Milanese Morning Custard (page 70). Contains peaches, ricotta cheese and yogurt. Serve with *Sesame Bread* (page 38). Contains whole wheat flour, unbleached white flour, sesame seeds, lemon peel, egg, milk, oil and honey.

LUNCH

Baby's Turnip and Carrot Dinner (page 83). Contains turnips, carrots, yogurt. Serve with *Bean-Bean Dinner* (page 53). Contains soybeans, green beans, pine nuts.

DINNER

Indian Eggplant Curry (page 136). Contains eggplant, potatoes, peppers, tomatoes, cloves, ginger, cinnamon. Serve with *Chilled Cranberry Soup* (page 155). Contains cranberries, oranges, lemon, banana, yogurt.

BEDTIME

The Basic Formula (page 89). Contains yeast, milk, banana.

Wednesday

BREAKFAST

Abby Van Derek's Incredible Granola (page 32), *with milk and strawberries*. Contains grains, fruits, nuts.

LUNCH

8 A.M. *Oranges* (page 70). Contains oranges, apricots, cereal, sunflower seeds.

DINNER

Apple Annie's Tomato Sauce and Soybean Casserole (page 113). Contains soybeans, cheese, broccoli, wheat germ, tomatoes, apples, onions. Serve with a puréed fresh fruit in season from your own area of the country.

BEDTIME

The Basic Formula (page 89). Contains yeast, milk, banana.

Thursday

BREAKFAST

Soy Pancakes with honey; sprinkle with ground walnuts (page 52). Serve with some puréed fresh fruits from your own area.

LUNCH

Yammy Do (page 80). Contains yams, figs, bulgur wheat, banana, egg yolk. Serve with *Soybean-Cheese Meal* (page 52). Contains soybeans, cheese.

DINNER

Arizona Eggplant (page 118). Contains eggplant, zucchini, mushrooms, ricotta cheese, onions, tomato sauce. Serve with *Apple Flip* (page 161). Contains apples, raisins, cinnamon.

BEDTIME

The Basic Formula (page 89). Contains yeast, milk, banana.

Friday

BREAKFAST

Abby Van Derek's Incredible Granola (page 32) with milk. Contains grains, fruits, nuts.

LUNCH
Pleasing Peas (page 85). Contains milk, peas, cheese, yogurt. Serve with *Simple Soybean Pulp* (page 51). Contains soybeans.

DINNER
Pistachio-Lentil Soup (page 158). Contains lentils, pistachio nuts, onions, carrots, tomato paste, cumin seed, turmeric. Serve with *Grace's Vegetables à la Mode* (page 128). Contains zucchini, onions, mushrooms, cheese, yogurt.

BEDTIME
The Basic Formula (page 89). Contains yeast, milk, banana.

Saturday

BREAKFAST
Winter Breakfast Pudding (page 65). Contains yogurt and apricots. Serve with toasted *Gig's Dill Bread* (page 36). Contains whole wheat flour, unbleached white flour, egg, dill weed, dill seed, cottage cheese.

LUNCH
Eastern Casserole (page 114). Contains lentils, rice, onions, peppers, nuts, cheese.

DINNER
Canyon de Chelly Casserole (page 123) with tossed green salad. Contains pinto beans, green chilis, tomatoes, Cheddar cheese.

BEDTIME
The Basic Formula (page 89). Contains yeast, milk, banana.

A NOTE ON INGREDIENTS

ADZUKI BEANS: These are small, red Japanese beans. When cooked, they have a rich, hearty, slightly sweet flavor, vaguely reminiscent of pinto beans. While not yet widely used in the United States, this bean has grown somewhat in popularity via its use in Zen macrobiotic cooking.

APRICOT CONCENTRATE: Apricots in highly concentrated, thick liquid form. This concentrate can be diluted with water to make apricot juice; or a teaspoon or so can be added to homemade yogurt or other foods to add a delicate flavor. Apricot and other fruit concentrates such as black cherry and blueberry are usually available in health-food stores. They are fairly expensive for casual use, but their compact size makes them convenient for a mother who must travel with a child.

BLACKSTRAP MOLASSES: A by-product of cane-sugar refining. This molasses is a rich source of iron. Combined with Tamari soy sauce as a seasoning for cooked dried beans, it is also a source of calcium.

GOAT'S MILK: Of all the animal milks, goat's milk is undoubtedly best for children. It is very digestible because the fat globules are integrated into the milk, not gathered on top. It is rich in calcium, fluorine and phosphorus. For these reasons, and because its consistency is similar to that of mother's milk, it is recommended for young babies, if for some reason the mother is unable to nurse—or when it is time to wean the child.

SEA SALT: The preferred seasoning salt, because in its natural state it contains iodine and all the trace minerals. Much of the other salt available today has been chemically treated.

SEAWEEDS: Among the many edible seaweeds are Hijiki, Nori and Agar-agar. Seaweeds are far richer in iodine than other foods, and 80 percent of this iodine is in a form most easily absorbed into the system. Seaweeds are also an excellent source of iron, other minerals, and the known trace minerals. These foods from the sea have long been used in Japanese cuisine and are beginning to be appreciated in ours. Dried, they can be purchased in Oriental markets, specialty and health-food shops.

SESAME SEA SALT (also called *Gomasio*): This combination of roasted unhulled sesame seeds and sea salt can be bought ready-made in health-food stores, but you can save money by making your own as follows: Roast 8 heaping tablespoons of unhulled sesame seeds over a medium flame, shaking the pan frequently and stirring the seeds around so that they brown evenly. When lightly browned and beginning to pop, remove from heat and grind together with 2 tablespoons of sea salt. This can be done with a mortar and pestle or in a blender. Store in an airtight jar. Use instead of plain sea salt on rice, noodles, salad, etc. Its rich nutlike flavor enhances many foods.

SOYBEAN OLEOMARGARINE: A margarine made from soybean oil, water, salt and finely ground soybeans. Packaged in the same manner as butter, it is carried by health-food stores and some specialty food shops. It is recommended as a replacement for butter in your child's diet from the very beginning.

SOYBEANS: One of the oldest crops of mankind. Soybean protein is of good quality and sufficiently complete to sustain life for a long period of time. Because soybeans contain only half the carbohydrates of other dried beans, and little starch, they are a good item in diabetic and starch-restricted diets. They may be introduced to your child at an early age—soybean puree can be digested as early as six to eight months. *Soybean milk*, like goat's milk, can be substituted for mother's milk, should this be necessary.

TAHINI: Ground sesame seed paste, available in health food, Greek and Turkish food stores.

TAMARI SOY SAUCE: "Tamari" is not a brand name; it denotes a naturally fermented soy sauce stored in wooden barrels for at least two years to age. It is made from water, soybeans, wheat and sea salt and is rich in natural sugars, oils, minerals and vitamins. Because of the unhurried aging process and freedom from chemical preservatives, it is slightly more expensive than other soy sauces, but well worth the extra cost. It can be bought in any health-food store.

TOFU: A delicately flavored, soft-textured soy bean curd. It also comes in smoked form. Tofu is available at Oriental food shops.

TUPELO HONEY: This honey, made from the nectar of tupelo-tree blossoms, is considered the most delicate and subtle of all honeys. Tupelo and other honeys are a primary source of energy; it is advisable to consider them the only sweetening your child ever gets on a regular basis.

WHEATBERRIES: The genesis of the wheat grain itself, these are both the seed and fruit of the shaft. From wheatberries come such products as wheat flour, wheat germ, bulgur and couscous. The berries can be sprouted in the same manner as soybeans. Wheatberry sprouts are good in tossed salads and sandwiches; steamed with other vegetables; or by themselves, seasoned with Tamari soy sauce and a little lemon juice.

If you have difficulty in obtaining any of the foods suggested throughout the recipes, the following health food distributors may be helpful for information on where they can be purchased:

Sherman Foods, Inc.
276 Jackson Avenue
Bronx, New York 10454

Balanced Foods, Inc.
2500 83 Street
North Bergen, New Jersey 07047

Mottel Health Foods, Inc.
451 Washington Street
New York, New York 10013

RECOMMENDED READINGS

*Nature's Children: A Guide to
Organic Foods and
Herbal Remedies for Children*
Juliette de Bairacli Levy
Schocken Books
1971; 146 pages.

Diet For A Small Planet
Frances Moore Lappe
Ballantine Books, Inc.
1971; 301 pages.

The Soybean Cookbook
Dorothea Van Gundy Jones
Arc Books
1963; 240 pages.

New Age Vegetarian Cookbook
The Rosicrucian Fellowship
1968; 492 pages.

Victory Through Vegetables
Joan Wiener and Barbara Thralls
Ballantine Books
1972; 178 pages.

The Natural Foods Cookbook
Beatrice Trum Hunter
Simon and Schuster
1961 (cloth); 296 pages.
1969 (paper); 296 pages.

Zen Cookery
Ohsawa Foundation, Inc.
The Ignoramus Press
1966; 79 pages.

The Gayelord Hauser Cookbook
Gayelord Hauser
Capricorn Books
1946; 312 pages.

Eating Your Way To Health
Dr. Max Bircher-Benner
Penguin Books
1972; 341 pages.

Yoga Natural Foods Cookbook
Richard Hittleman
Bantam Books
1970; 160 pages.

WHEN TO FEED BABY WHAT

The recipes below are gathered into groups according to the time when baby is first ready for these foods.

RECOMMENDED FOR PREGNANT WOMEN

Asian Garden Salad, 27
Bel Paese Soufflé, 24
Between Meals, 24
Breakfast Drink, Daily, 24
Custard, Baby, 168
Peppers, Mama's Stuffed, 26
Raisin Shake, 92
Raisin Yogurt, Miss Ann's, 73
Yogurt Dessert, 28

RECOMMENDED FOR BABY

From birth:
Dried Milk, 32
Soybean Milk, 32
Yogurt, 31

From three months on:
Breakfast Pudding, Winter, 65
Brown Rice, Steamed, 42
First Meal (Fruits), 64
Rice for Baby, Mushy, 42
Soybeans, Cooked, 41

From four months on:
Dutch Dinner Vegetables, 141
Yams, Basic Baked, or Sweet Potatoes, 80
Yam Pone Poke, 80

From four to six months on:
Accord Summer Drink, 104
Apricot Malt, 103
Apricot November, 103
Autumn Lunch, 74
Baby's Dinner Soufflé, 84
Blue Plate Special, 76
Blueberry Summer Cooler, 101
Breakfast, Very Easy, 63
Breakfast, Working Baby, 93
Breakfast-Plus Booster Drink, 97
Bright and Early, 104
Cantaloupe Drink, Cool, 99
Cranberries, Cooked, 65
December Morning Quickie, 98
Dinner Divine, 74
Early One Morning, 102
Early September, 93
Figs à la Barrow Street, 72
Funny Dinner, 71
Grape Drink, Grand, 102